FASCIA
DECOMPRESSION
The Missing Link in Self-Care

FASCIA
DECOMPRESSION
The Missing Link in Self-Care

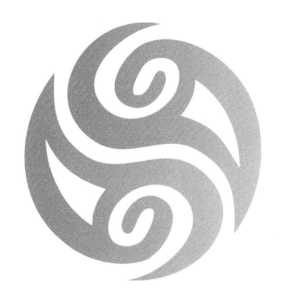

Deanna Hansen

Copyright
© July 2019
All Rights Reserved
Published by Fluid Isometrics
Winnipeg, Manitoba Canada

No part of this work may be used or reproduced, transmitted, stored or used in any form or by any means graphic, electronic, or mechanical, including but not limited to photocopying, recording, scanning, digitizing, distribution, information networks or information storage and retrieval systems, or in any manner whatsoever without prior written permission.

For further information, contact info@fluidisometrics.com

Printed in the United States and Canada

Cover Design and Interior Design and Formatting by

www.emtippettsbookdesigns.com

Disclaimer

This book contains information that is intended to help the readers be better informed consumers of health care. It is presented as general advice on health care. Always consult your doctor for your individual needs.

Before beginning any new exercise program, it is recommended that you seek medical advice from your personal physician.

This book is not intended to be a substitute for the medical advice of a licensed physician. The reader should consult with their doctor in any matters relating to his/her health.

Table of Contents

Prologue 1

Chapter 1: The Awakening 5

Chapter 2: The Seeds 12

Chapter 3: Size Loss/Space Gain 17

Chapter 4: Understanding Pain 22

Chapter 5: Injury-A Different Approach 29

Chapter 6: Aging Has a Pattern 38

Chapter 7: Cellular Migration 44

Chapter 8: What You Think You Become 52

Chapter 9: Building Foundations 59

Chapter 10: The Healing Crisis 69

Chapter 11: Another Foundation-The Power of the Tongue 75

Chapter 12: Aligning the Ribcage-An Essential Component for Health ... 81

Chapter 13: Introducing Block Therapy 88

Chapter 14: Following the Flow 97

Epilogue: A Brighter Future 106

About the Author 111

Introduction

Understanding Fascia and Block Therapy

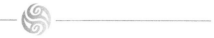

What actually causes aging? We know it can be seen in the lines of our face, the spots on our skin, the thinning of our hair and the sagging, hanging tissue that was once taut and firm. It is also the degeneration of our body's tissue resulting in pain and disease. The ultimate driver of this is gravity. Simply, as we go through time, we decrease in our internal space; we get shorter and wider as we age; we compress. The constant force of gravity is relentless at pulling down on the body. We don't even recognize this force and how it acts on the cells because it is always present.

The good news: we have an anti-gravity design built right in.

It all comes down to understanding the fascia system. Fascia is the tissue connecting every one of our hundred trillion cells -- like a 3-dimensional fishnet. In fact, I see the fascia as being the cell membrane of every cell, connected to every other cell.

For fascia to be healthy and supportive to the body, it needs to be at a certain temperature. Fascia tubules are hollow and filled with liquid, and they carry light. This means messages can travel through the fascia at the speed of light. This is incredibly important to understand for health. If the fascia becomes thick or cold, transmissions are affected.

When transmissions are affected, body, mind and spirit are compromised. Physical, mental and emotional health all require steady flow to accept the incoming information from the external world, and to release the debris, byproducts of functioning, toxins, negative emotion, and stuck patterns of thinking. A compressed frozen body is a body out of balance and the whole of our being suffers from it.

It is through proper mechanics of the body that we maintain the optimal tissue temperature. The diaphragm muscle is situated in the core of the body, acting as the ceiling to the abdominal organs and the floor to the heart and lungs. When we inhale, the muscle moves down in the core and the belly extends; when we exhale, the muscle moves up and the belly squeezes small. Breathing with the diaphragm muscle is like turning on the furnace in the body. This muscle's action regulates the core temperature with its continual movement up and down through proper inhalation and exhalation. Correct posture is required to support the diaphragm's shape and action. When we collapse into the core from unconscious posture, the diaphragm doesn't have the opportunity to move in the way in which it is designed.

When the diaphragm can't function, the muscles of the upper chest kick in to pull in the breath, but this is limiting to the health of the fascia as the overall temperature of the body becomes cooler. If breathing with the diaphragm is like turning on the furnace, breathing with the chest muscles is like putting a space heater in a room. Only that room will be heated, not the whole building.

Not only does the lack of movement from the diaphragm affect tissue temperature, but tissue compression from incorrect posture also causes cooling. Tissue needs space in order for fluids to travel freely. Compressed tissue is dense and creates roadblocks, or tree trunks of restriction. For tissue to be healthy and clean, it needs to have room for blood and oxygen to reach each and every cell, and to clean them of debris. We need to de-compress tissue manually in order to remove the roadblocks, and heat the tissue with the full conscious breath.

In Gil Headly's "Fuzz Speech", he shares that "fuzz" consists of adhesions that develop between the layers of fascia from lack of movement and cooling of the system. The older "fuzz" can become very thick to the point where a scalpel is required to move through it. This would be fascia in deep freeze. Thick, frozen fascia needs to be decompressed and heated to liquefy the fluids and promote movement and freedom.

Block Therapy is incredibly efficient at heating and liquefying -- melting adhesions. Block Therapy is a self-care practice that uses a tool called the Block Buddy. A person lies over the Block Buddy in various positions throughout the body for a minimum of 3 minutes. This creates pressure in the areas, which stimulates circulation. Through the practice of diaphragmatic breathing, the body's internal furnace is switched on, creating an increase in the overall temperature of the fascia. The combination of external pressure from the Block Buddy and diaphragmatic breath effectively melts the adhesions to promote optimal flow throughout the entire body.

Understanding the mechanics of cellular health can be overwhelming, but really it is simple if you understand the fascia and its role. There is a lot of confusion out there because it is only recently that attention has been given to the fascia system. Simply put, fascia needs to be properly aligned so fluids can travel freely. When there are blocks from compression and a cooling from incorrect breathing, flow to and from cells is compromised. We accept aging as a normal fact of life. Pain, aging and disease are realities we face and deal with as the need arises. However, there is an approach that will turn back the hands of time and take your tissue in the opposite direction from compression. Block Therapy puts back into the tissue the space that time and gravity have taken away. It decompresses!

I look forward in the following pages to sharing my journey and the many testimonials of individuals who practice Block Therapy. The best part about Block Therapy is that if you do it, you understand it. The proof is in the practice.

Breathe & Believe

Shelley Elhatton

I will never forget how I first came to hear about Block Therapy. It was a very dark time in my life. After a lifetime of working full time as a nurse, always caring for others, I found myself on disability. I was in chronic constant pain, unable to walk properly. Sitting was also so hard, and getting up from seated to standing was incredibly difficult. I couldn't do life as I once did.

Specialists after specialists and MRIs after MRIs, and still no diagnosis for all the pain I was experiencing. That summer day sitting on my deck I was so frustrated. I loved to garden -- gardening is such a passion -- but I couldn't even pull a weed! I sat there crying. Well, it was more like sobbing and praying to whoever would hear me.

I always believed that the body, if given what it needed, could heal. I had tried everything that I knew as a nurse with a holistic background, yet I was still in so much pain. I was so depressed and started thinking maybe all of this was just in my head...was I creating this?

It was that very next day, sharing time with a friend over a coffee, that she asked, "Have you ever heard of Block Therapy, created by Deanna Hansen?" Interestingly enough, I had heard of her; I was receiving her emails, yet hadn't read any of them. When my friend said " Block Therapy", it really resonated with me. I was beyond interested.

We looked up the classes and registered that very day. We both had no idea what it was all about. We brought our yoga mats and attended our first class. Little did I know, this was the beginning of a new life -- a much healthier way of life.

As I lay on my mat, with this hand crafted wooden block, I listened very intently. We focused on our breath. I was breathing in a way different than I had before. It is called diaphragmatic breathing. Deanna spoke so fluently. She was a wealth of knowledge.

This system called fascia was the missing piece to why our bodies get sick. It just made so much sense to me. I have been a nurse forever, and as a nurse I always wondered why he or she got sick instead of that other person…as she spoke, I could see the body, the inside of the body, and I got it!

No wonder I was sick and in so much pain!! All those years of doing all those repetitive movements and all my childhood injuries, plus surgeries, all add up to the perfect internal storm!!

I felt amazing after that first class! I still didn't really understand, but what I heard made sense. I knew and trusted that my body was happy, and that I needed this.

As shy as I was and as much as I wanted to stay invisible to the world (I had gained so much weight) I needed to go meet this Deanna and tell her how I was feeling and how much I needed to learn this work so I could heal myself, and then go help others like me to heal also.

Deanna and I are now very good friends. I feel so blessed to have her in my life. Making the decision to attend a class and embrace this work has been a life-changing gift.

I was slow at first, then I began a daily practice. The Teacher Training program really helped me see the body and its dis-ease in a different way. The fascia system is amazing and connects us from head to toe.

I returned to work part time after a year of starting on the block. Today, my life is so busy and full. I amaze myself at what I can do now; I am so strong and flexible. I love to teach and share what I have learned as a teacher and nurse.

Thank you Deanna for bringing this practice to the world. It truly is life-changing!

Much Love

Prologue

It was the turn of the century. I was 30 years old and in my second "failed" marriage. I remember asking my sister if there was anything wrong with me. She said, "All that matters is whether you are happy".

That was a profound statement, I had always worried about everyone else's happiness, never my own. I realized in that moment that I needed to take a good long look at myself and make some changes.

I am extreme in my behavior and personality. At times this has been a gift, at others a curse. For years, my extreme nature was getting the better of me. Finally, I found an "addiction" that would change not only my life, but the lives of many others.

The Birth of Fluid Isometrics

For about 5 years, for 5 hours a day, I was diving into my own tissue with my hands, exploring my body. It started in my abdomen, where I spent most of my time in the beginning, and gradually evolved to embrace all areas. I continued to discover things about myself with each passing sweep of the hand. Along the way I was learning different textures and sensations, and experiencing an array of changes. The effects were endless, and all positive.

Imagine: for 5 years, every day, I would spend hours working in my tissue, the rest of the day treating patients with a skill I seemed to be channeling. About 2 years into this routine, a patient said I should be teaching my technique. It was the first time anyone had suggested such a thing, and I realized I wasn't even sure what I was doing. I was following some unseen energy that was guiding my hands, and people were experiencing amazing results.

There definitely was something guiding me; it wasn't some intellectual creation. I always say to people, "I didn't develop Fluid Isometrics, it developed me". And that was and is the beauty of it. There was something so compelling about the process and sensations that I couldn't help myself.

In the beginning, relief from anxiety was the draw; but very quickly it became about weight loss/shape shifting. I couldn't believe it: I had spent years trying to force my body to lose weight and change its shape, but with all my efforts I was getting bigger and experiencing more pain. I was 50 pounds overweight and nothing was working for me. It was incredibly discouraging.

To have found something so simple that was getting the results I had struggled for in vain was groundbreaking. Literally, the answer I had been seeking was at my fingertips. Little did I know how this would ultimately dominate my life; but here I am, and I wouldn't dream of doing anything else.

As I mentioned, my focus for a long time was on my abdomen. This wasn't a conscious choice; it felt right. The 50 extra pounds I was carrying seemed to be centered in my core, which was a place of extreme self-loathing. I had always envied women with beautiful hourglass figures. I actually believed that if I had the belly I desired I would never feel stress.

It wasn't just vanity. Large a factor as that was, it wasn't the principal reason I so obsessively hated this area. It felt ugly. There was a combination of feelings and sensations surrounding it that made me profoundly unhappy. Now I know that one of the main reasons was that I was filled with waste. How can we feel beautiful and sexy with years of undigested food and waste trapped inside us?

I also couldn't move with the freedom I desired. Because I was so compacted and compressed, my movements were labored and awkward. All I wanted was to be free. My ability to express myself was trapped in the folds of tissue that weighed me down. It was as if gravity had imprisoned the carefree child I once had been.

With so much negative emotion attached to my core, it wasn't long before I awakened to the amazing benefits I was experiencing while intuitively working in my abdomen. In fact, it only took a couple of days to see the changes in my size and shape. After only the second time I did this self-work, when I stood up, I felt different. I went to the mirror to look at myself and immediately began to cry. I had found the solution to years of pain and anguish.

Chapter 1

The Awakening

I had just left my second husband. I was also going through a painful business separation. For years I had been using alcohol to numb the stress, but I had been sober for a few months and the anxiety was ramping up. One particular evening, I was flurrying in the worst anxiety attack I had ever known. It was absolutely terrifying. I'm sure many of you have experienced this: being frozen with fear. I felt paralyzed, stuck in a dizzying vortex of guilt and shame. For a moment, I thought I might die; I couldn't breathe.

Then it happened.

I dove my hand into my belly. It wasn't a conscious act; it was a reaction to not breathing. That initial plunge triggered an exhalation filled with pain and fear, straight from the core, that cleared the way for breath, for life. I sucked in the air as though I had come up from under water, and got ahold of myself. In that moment, I gained control.

The first sensation I encountered was pain. Stark in its intensity, it was equally profound in its effect. The pain took me to the exhalation. It took me to the place I had been afraid of, and it pushed itself through the barrier. It punctured a seal I had created over years of struggle, and gave me access to a center of pure calm.

I continued to explore. The relief I felt was so impacting that I wanted to prolong it indefinitely. I combined adding pressure into my abdomen with exhaling deeply, and felt incredible relief. I was moving the fear, the thoughts of the past, the stuck emotion, purposefully out of my being. With each new breath I felt lighter and cleaner.

You can't imagine the sensations running through me at that time. I had spent years and years trying to force my body to be what I wanted it to be, with frustratingly opposite results. Not only was I bigger than I wanted to be; my tissue felt hard, cold and dense. I was weighty, and it affected my movements. Everything was labored and painful.

The realization that I had discovered something that would remove the internal pressure inspired such enthusiasm that I couldn't stop the work. Every day, after spending 8-10 hours on patients, I would come home and spend my remaining waking time exploring my own tissue. It was as if I had started a magical journey where every corner I turned revealed new gifts and treasures.

I remember one night having dinner with a friend. An area in my pectoralis muscle had caught my attention, and as we were sitting at dinner, I proceeded to dive my hand into my shirt. There in public, as we were conversing, I was spiraling my hand into my chest. He said, " do you think you can not do this right now?" I had been doing it so regularly it had become automatic. It was what I did; I stopped, but the second I got back into the car, I was at it again.

Not only was the work improving my mental and emotional state; the physical changes were miraculous.

At the age of 22 I had breast reduction surgery. Prior to that, whenever I put on weight, it went to my breasts and belly: I felt like a balloon ready to burst. I remember seeing a woman who was flat chested and didn't need a bra, and envying her. To be free of that fullness, that heaviness, that burden, would be a dream. Looking back, I am pleased I had the surgery. It was a huge improvement to the quality of my life. I could finally buy a regular bra and properly fit into clothes. Most of all, I didn't feel self-conscious about my size.

The surgery left a long scar underneath each breast. As the years passed I noticed the scar was building in size and seemed to restrict my breathing. I didn't know that that was a factor in my asthma symptoms until I created changes to the scar tissue years after I began the self-work. Today, knowing what I know, I wouldn't choose surgery on purpose; but it created an opportunity for me to work on the scars that had actually sealed themselves to my ribs.

I have put countless hours into exploring the area and observing the results. Awhile into the practice I noticed a loosening in the tissue that made it easier to move. As it was my ribs I was working on, my breathing became easier. I even stopped using my asthma inhaler, something that had become a bit of a crutch before a run. I was able to take much more air into my lungs when exercising, and could lift my ribcage up and back, standing taller and straighter every day. My breasts changed as well; I was rebuilding their foundation, and they were lifting with time.

It was a very interesting process. I had the opportunity to feel the tissue sensations with my hands, and associated pain I was tapping into, then apply that awareness to helping my patients. Because I knew what the tissue texture felt like, it was easy to know what my patients were feeling. I also became aware of their breathing patterns.

As I mentioned at the beginning, connecting the exhalation to the pain creates space in tissue to bring in oxygen. I knew from Yoga training and my own experience that pain, fear and stress cause us to hold our breath. This meant that, where my work on my patients involved pain, until I taught them how to breathe it out, the benefits would be limited. That became a pivotal point in understanding the process.

Gradually I realized that what I was doing was putting space, therefore blood flow, back into areas of my body that were compressed. My hard, frozen belly was becoming flatter, calmer looking, warmer to the touch, and freer in its movement.

Before, when I was working so hard to change my shape, I would go for five mile runs, do Tae-Bo and aerobics, and, although dripping with sweat, find many areas on my body ice cold: notably my abdomen. It would drive me crazy because that was the area I most wanted to change. When I dove my hand into it that first night, the night of my anxiety attack, I felt not only pain, but also scar tissue.

Once I caught my breath and got past the initial sensations, I noticed that the area felt marbled. This didn't make sense. I hadn't had any injuries or surgeries there, yet it felt the same as the scar tissue I massaged every day in patients.

Then it hit me: why all those years of hard work had accomplished nothing. This compressed, dense tissue was acting as a barrier to blood flow. How could I possibly metabolize fat if the blood couldn't get to it? It needed to be decompressed, and that is exactly what was happening with this intuitive process.

The forty-five minutes I spent working on myself that first night were magical. It was amazing how I was awakening to tissue sensations I hadn't known; equally fascinating was the information I was uncovering. As I would drag my hand through the tissue, different layers of density would present themselves, sharing some past event and the emotion attached. Right away, something felt right on a really deep level. I felt I had found a way finally take control of my body.

Kristine Wattis

My name is Kristine Wattis. I started Block Therapy back in September of 2013. I didn't know what I was getting into as no one I knew was doing it at that time. I received a flyer in the mail and read it. It was a simple flyer showing Deanna holding a block of wood, and it listed the benefits of Block Therapy. Back then there was no website where I could find out more information, so all I could go on was what I found on Deanna Hansen. I ended up reading an e-book she wrote called "The Power of Conscious Breathing". Something in that book resonated with me and I decided to try Block Therapy.

It's been the best thing I've ever done in regards to my health. I was hooked after the first class. I thought that this therapy needed to be shouted from the rooftops. That was my exact thought. I immediately shared it with members of my family.

I noticed soon after starting Block Therapy how my breathing improved. At the time I would not have thought that my breathing was restricted in any way as I never suffered from allergies or lung problems. To me, my breathing was normal. However, once I started using the block, melting through the adhesions of fascia solidifying my ribs, and applying the postural recommendations in Block Therapy, I realized that I wasn't really breathing properly before. I was now breathing deeper, fuller breaths and it felt great!

I also used to experience debilitating back pain at least once a year since I was 18. It usually happened in the springtime. I would literally have to walk hunched over, because otherwise there would be too much pain, which lasted for about a week. My doctor would prescribe muscle relaxants that would provide some relief. Since starting Block Therapy I have not had this debilitating back pain. All with no use of drugs of any sort. I love that natural healing aspect of Block Therapy. There is no more reaching for a bottle of pills; rather I reach for my block to address any issue I may be feeling at the time.

In 2016 I joined the Block Therapy University Teacher Training program to learn all there is to know about Block Therapy. Little did I know that the community I was joining is one of the best, supportive communities out there, led by Deanna Hansen!

I'm now a Block Therapy Instructor, sharing it with as many people as I can. There's no better feeling than when you are able to help others, and I thank Deanna for bringing her dream to life and giving it to the rest of us to share.

BLOCK ON!

Chapter 2

The Seeds

I come from a family in which appearance, particularly weight, was a major preoccupation. As a kid, I had a skinny, agile, naturally athletic body, but when puberty struck my cells ballooned. My size seemed to accumulate around my middle. Wanting to reset my body back to a time when I had control, I slipped easily into an unhealthy eating pattern.

Being self-conscious about my middle, I worked to make my abdomen as tight and strong as possible to hold in the ever-expanding tissue. This is one of those folk practices that I have learned has dire consequences: "Hold your stomach in". I'm sure most of you have heard or done this but the reality is that doing it stops you from breathing! Not entirely, of course. The body is ingenious in its design. If one of its functions is impeded, it finds another way to fulfill it. When our abdominal muscles are continually contracted, the diaphragm muscle freezes and we begin to pull in air with the muscles of the upper chest.

When I think about it now I want to choke. Recalling the sensation of forcing an unnatural muscular action, and knowing how much harm I was causing, makes me sad. The worst part was that I lost my connection to my body. But that is what happened -- puberty hit me like a truck and I started to disconnect from myself. I had gained twenty pounds and acquired hips and breasts seemingly overnight.

I remember getting my first bra. This was not a good time in my life. The sense of expanding in all these different directions made me feel out of control, and now I had to wear a sling to hold back this renegade flesh. I was in the department store, wanting to be anywhere but. I grabbed the first bra I saw and went to the changing room to try it on.

It was so tight I almost couldn't do it up. I felt my temperature rising and wanted to scream. The thought of having to try on a bunch of these sent me into panic mode. I told the clerk it fit, and this was what I took home.

I had to babysit that night. I put on the bra and walked down the street, suffocating from the tension. By the time I put the kids to bed, I just had to take the evil contraption off. I sat there bawling my eyes out as I realized I was in for a prison sentence. I was trapped in someone else's body and I hated it. However, I had to get used to wearing this thing.

I put the bra back on, feeling exhausted and scared. I tried to maneuver my ribcage so I could squeeze in a little more of myself. I found that if I took the shallowest breaths, I could manage it for a while. And so began a breathing pattern based in fear and starvation, one that dramatically affected my entire physical, mental and emotional life.

Remembering these moments as I was diving into my tissue made me feel both sad and relieved. Sad because it brought me back to that scared, disconnected girl. Relieved because it was all starting to make sense. When I hit a hard and compact area, I would linger and let myself feel what my fingertips were sensing. What I noticed was that if I waited and focused on exhaling, the area would open up and become softer and warmer. This would bring a release of tension, lightness to the tissue, and greater range and flexibility to my movements.

It also made it easier to breathe. As I played around in the area, I was able to expand my belly more, taking in more oxygen with each breath. As I mentioned earlier, after only the second day of this work I stood up and felt remarkably different: taller. My tissue looked flatter and calmer than it had in years.

It's pretty awesome really. The diaphragm muscle is the one designed to pull air into the lungs to acquire the oxygen that feeds the entire body. It also functions to exhale the carbon dioxide and other waste. The beauty of this lies in the fact that the majority of the alveoli (oxygen receptor sites) are concentrated at the base of the lungs. So when we breathe with the diaphragm, air gets pulled deeply enough into the lungs to reach this bed of abundance. When we walk around holding our bellies in, we are forcing an unnatural breathing pattern, thereby starving ourselves of the most vital nutrient for life.

As I came to understand how cells respond to breathing, it became clear to me why my abdomen was do dense. The weakened diaphragm's inability to support the ribcage and inflate its cells properly had resulted in dense and heavy tissue. Being an unconscious breather, neglecting the diaphragm muscle, had resulted in a collapse of the entire ribcage into the core, displacing my abdomen and its contents outward.

With this newfound understanding, I felt empowered. I already knew that if I continued this process, the positive benefits would carry on.

Lorraine Knoroski

The Power of Block Therapy

After doing Block Therapy for over 3 years, the changes I experience continue to surprise me. I love that I no longer deal with TMJ pain or aggravating shoulder pain and tension. I love that I am no longer plagued with digestive issues like bloating, stomach pain and sleepless nights spent sitting upright in bed. I'm relieved the twinge in my back that used to stop me in my tracks is gone, the constant ache and swelling in a damaged finger is gone, and my wrist pain is gone and kept at bay with the practice of BT.

My varicose veins are dramatically reduced and my eczema is a thing of the past. The tightness in my throat with difficulty swallowing that plagued me for years pre - and post - surgery is a thing of the past. Tinnitus is reduced substantially and ocular migraines are all but eliminated. Feelings of anxiety are under my control through diaphragmatic breathing.

Since bringing Block Therapy into daily practice, I enjoy increased energy and endurance and a greater fluidity in movement. In spite of aging, I have been told I have a younger looking appearance, thicker hair, better posture, and a greater symmetry in my body. My eyelids are more open; droopy eyelids are gone.

My double chin is gone and my jaw line is cleaner looking. My concentration has also improved.

All this has been accomplished entirely without surgery or medication, just this beautiful self-care practice called Block Therapy. I love the renewed health and happiness BT brings me. Block Therapy is a practice available to people of all ages and abilities and allows each individual to have their own personal control and improve their health at their own pace.

Chapter 3

Size Loss/Space Gain

I certified as an athletic therapist at the age of 24. I knew from my education what I was supposed to do to have a healthy body; yet that goal eluded me. Something didn't make sense. I understood that to lose weight we have to ingest less energy than we expend. But this rule didn't seem to apply to me.

How frustrating to spend hours every day, doing weights, running laps, eating little, and still getting big. Not only was my body looking anything but attractive; I was feeling like a total failure. I grew to hate my body. If only I looked different, I thought everything wrong in my life would be fixed. Yet here I was, trapped in an alternate universe where the laws of weight loss didn't apply.

How many of you work really hard to lose weight only to fail continually? Weight loss is something so many are seeking yet aren't achieving. Part of the reason is that we are not looking at the most efficient solution. Maybe if we changed the focus, we would approach our mission in a different way.

There are only two times in our life when we actually increase the number of fat cells in the body: when we are babies; and when we hit puberty. Otherwise, if our size is increasing, it is because the fat cells are expanding. So what makes them expand?

When we breathe consciously and practise proper posture, we keep the cells in the body intact and in their appropriate positions. When we don't, the chest literally collapses into the core of the body, taking away our inner space and limiting the diaphragm's ability to function. The result is a displacement of tissue outward, also known as bulging belly and love handles. This is why it is harder to "lose weight" as we get older. It isn't the weight we should be trying to lose; it is the internal space we should be focused on gaining.

I honestly don't know where I would be now had I not found a way to breathe life back in. Depression started taking me down. The years between 20-30 were particularly painful and dark and the effects had taken hold of my every moment. I don't believe that in that entire decade there was a single time when I was fully present. I lived in a world of guilt, shame, self-loathing, and wishing to be anyone but who I was. Every day I thank God for that fateful moment -- the anxiety attack when this all began.

The understanding was immediate. By the second day of my self-work, I knew I had the solution. Every day I would come home from work, put on some music, and resume this personal exploration. As I would soften the dense tissue with my hands and expand the area with my breath, I found I could exhale more fully and efficiently. This meant that I could make my belly look smaller.

Somewhere along the way it struck me: rather than hold the stomach in, we need to squeeze the belly small. The idea of making the abdomen large with the inhalation and small with the exhalation brought a whole new understanding to me. At first it felt very wrong, making my belly big on purpose, but I quickly learned that the combined massage and controlled use of the diaphragm muscle was changing the shape of my core.

People started commenting that I was looking better. I started to understand that aligning the tissue properly was more important than literal weight loss. I could feel and see the release of weight and tension, and the quality of my tissue was improving in general. I had a different perspective that made total sense and was actually working.

My waist was getting smaller, my arms were getting toned and sculpted, my legs felt and looked better, and my face had cleaner contours. I started to see that posture mattered when it came to how the tissue compressed and ballooned. As I would release tension in the belly with my hands, I found it was easier to stand straighter. Be as tall as you can was my mantra, and every day I worked, I noticed a greater ease in sitting and standing upright.

Another negative consequence that happens when we "fall in" to our core is that we block proper digestion and elimination. When the diaphragm muscle is working, it gives the abdominal organs a continual massage, keeping them heated and functioning. When it isn't, these organs become cold and consequently function less efficiently. This causes a sluggish system where food isn't digested properly and waste isn't eliminated fully and completely. This results in bloating, weight gain and pain.

My Nanny, my Mom's Mom, lived with us until I was nine, when she passed away. She was from the farm and used to bake her own bread, juice vegetables, make granola and feed me prunes. After she passed, my diet changed and over the years my ability to eliminate efficiently became increasingly problematic.

It's amazing how not releasing waste can dominate your mind. Whether I was going to have a decent day depended on 2 things: what the scale said, and whether I had had a bowel movement. If the number on the scale was high or I was blocked, the stress would suffocate me and the pressure would build. I remember looking at myself on such a day: I looked red, as if I was ready to explode.

Being of fair complexion, I also struggled with rosacea. My cheeks were always red and I had a lot of broken blood vessels. The first time I had a facial the esthetician was shocked at the amount of damage to my skin. I now understand the reason: my cells were under immense pressure and were full of toxins because I wasn't breathing properly.

Thankfully, as I continued on my path, everything started to change. Clothes were feeling looser; waste was leaving my body; and the numbers on the scale were changing rapidly. In addition there was a change in the color of my skin -- it looked calmer and healthier. Another blessing!

Victoria Goodman

I just knew, right from the beginning, that Block Therapy would deliver great results. I had a rotator cuff injury, not better after 3 years, so I decided to test Deanna's theory on my sore shoulder and never looked back!

In less than 2 years, I have transformed my body, from suffering in pain to freedom from pain. I have slimmed down by 20 lbs or more, and toned and realigned my body! I have healed from shoulder pain, neck pain and restriction, carpal tunnel syndrome, headaches, brain fog, constipation, circulation problems, wrinkles, scar tissue, foot pain -- it even controls my hot flashes. I have increased energy and productivity!

I look and feel better NOW than before I had kids!

Thank you Deanna for giving me the Solution to All my Problems!

Forever Grateful,

Chapter 4

Understanding Pain

After about 2 weeks of my new regimen something else had changed: my chronic back pain was gone.

When I was a student in Athletic Therapy we had to do twelve hundred hours of clinical and field work. Massage is one of the modalities we are trained in, and I was particularly good at it. I had a knack for sensing and breaking down scar tissue. As a result, my supervisor always sent the athletes and regular patients to me for massage.

Once I certified, that quickly became the focus of my treatments. I developed a successful practice as people enjoyed the strength of my hands and the relief they were experiencing. But years of bending over a massage table resulted in chronic and at times extreme back pain.

I remember precisely the moment I realized I had no pain. It had always been there, every step, every movement, and then this one day I got to work and it was gone. I was shocked. I wasn't expecting anything like this and I couldn't believe it. The relief didn't last the whole day, but the fact that it had occurred excited me immensely.

It was on this day that I first told one of my regular patients what I was doing and the effect it was having. On impulse I asked if I could work in his abdomen the way I had been in my own. He jumped at the opportunity. It was fascinating exploring the area; interesting, after having spent only two weeks working on myself, to feel that same tissue density in my patient. When he stood up after the treatment, he smiled. He said it felt different.

Thus began a whole new method of treatment. I didn't understand exactly what I was doing, but what I did to myself, I did to my patients. And just as I was excited about what my own body was experiencing, my patients were sharing their success with me, and with others. Soon there wasn't enough time in the day to accommodate all these people. They were coming in droves.

About two years into the practice someone said I should be teaching it. With the demand for my services now greater than I could manage, I recognized the wisdom in her suggestion. I started to pay attention to the intuitive pattern my hands were following.

At the time I was deeply involved in the practice of Iyengar Yoga. I was in fact in the teacher training program. I was fortunate to have had an exceptional teacher the first time I tried it and I caught the bug. Among other things, it was teaching me about conscious breathing and alignment -- a natural fit for what I was learning intuitively through my work.

Iyengar Yoga is highly disciplined when it comes to alignment. I would go to class, learn the posture, and feel where I was restricted. Then I would go home, work on that area, and the following week would have acquired a deeper access to the posture. I didn't really think about this until a couple of years into the program. I would see people who had started when I did, who hadn't progressed in their postures even though they practiced regularly. My own approach was to find the limitation, take my hands to the dense tissue, breathe life and freedom into the area, and move to a deeper level.

It was starting to come together in my mind. The dense tissue that restricts movement and flow wasn't changing with the practice of Yoga alone, but was changing quickly when the postures were combined with tissue work and breathing. Every week I was becoming more flexible; before long I could move and contort my body in ways that others couldn't.

Yoga and stretching are great because they take your attention to what stops you from moving. If you are trying to do the splits, you go only as far as you can. Pain is generally the limiting factor in how we move, or how we don't move.

Think of a baby. With ease you can take a leg and move it behind the head. There seems to be nothing stopping the action. Imagine being able to do that to yourself, no matter what your age.

Breathe Life Into Your Fascia

Unless you are a gymnast or contortionist, few people can perform this action. So what changes?

Driven by gravity, the collapse of the body and the thickening of tissue over time create a sticky mess that clogs and traps waste. Where tissue sticks and glues to bone, it inhibits range of motion. This isn't typically where the pain is felt; pain is where the tension resides -- usually a distance away from the cause site.

Imagine someone pulling on your arm consistently. Over time, your shoulder would get tired and start to ache. Working on the shoulder may feel good in the moment, but to release the tension would require that the person let go of your arm. This is what was becoming obvious to me over time with the process.

I saw this in myself. The chronic back pain I had had for years was beginning to lessen, not from working on my back, but from working in my belly. I began to understand how the collapse from years of unconscious posture and breathing was creating a thick and compressed area in my pelvis.

This, by the way, was another site of particular dissatisfaction in my body. I had no butt, but I had a thick lower belly. As I was releasing this area with the work, it too began to change and look more aesthetically pleasing. Gradually, I was piecing things together and making sense of them. I knew that if I was going to teach this I needed to be able to explain how it worked.

Barry Gibson

"A block of wood? Are you kidding me?" A lifetime of struggling with back pain, mobility issues, negativity and fear, melted away by Block Therapy and that piece of wood!

I remember vividly when I was introduced to the block a few years ago. My wife and I were at a friend's and someone there had a block and was getting into this new seemingly strange therapy called Block Therapy. I was struggling mightily again with back pain and was desperate enough to give it a try. Of course I did it all wrong. Lying on it on my back, thinking that was the way, because all my other therapies focused on the back, almost killed me; I could barely get up from that piece of wood that first time, but was intrigued.

So was my wife, as she had some long term nagging sports related injuries that were not getting any better. We were intrigued enough thankfully to follow up quickly with Deanna Hansen and her "blocks of wood" therapy. I was skeptical, but desperate. After meeting with Deanna relief was fast -- not overnight, but it made sense, and positive changes were quick. She was the first therapist to actually deal with the causal problems, not the pain site. She's different, unique, just like Block Therapy -- so unique, so helpful. Once you get into it, it makes so much sense, I had one of those "ah hah" moments for my back pain, and have not looked back since.

My background: I'm a PGA of Canada Golf Professional who suffered most of his adult life with daily pain and mobility issues.

All from a lifetime of traumas, sports injuries, lifestyle and general repetitive golf motion strain, which culminated in the classic golfer lumbar L5-S1 disk herniation. All the years prior to that injury, no one could solve or explain my general pain and mobility issues. I was told it was just stiffness, genetics, injury, and plain old getting old -- general mechanical dysfunction, whatever that is. It all got way worse way more quickly after the disk injury. I had a couple of years following that of constant sciatic pain; sitting, standing, walking, resting, sleeping, general life, was painful -- never mind trying to play golf!

The continual back stiffness, lower back compression and pain were wearing me out. I was aging fast, putting on weight fast, and carrying around that huge extra weight of negative emotion and fear. Living with prolonged pain and injury is like living with a slow poison in your system that drains you of life. All the physical therapies and training I did, from chiro to physio to yoga to sports training and exercise, provided temporary relief but nothing lasting -- until Block Therapy.

Fast forward a few years. My daily pain is gone, without medication of any kind, not even over the counter stuff, or my big crutch: self medicating with too much alcohol. So grateful for a different way to live. I've gone from a ballooning 38-inch waist to now pushing a 32-inch waist, like when I was 30! I feel and look 20 years younger, and I'm 25 pounds lighter! I am able to live relatively pain free now, and all that negative baggage and fear I carried around for years has been released through the help of Block Therapy.

None of this was an overnight sensation, but results began to happen very quickly, and the block is now part of my daily living. It *compliments everything I do, and it's not a huge time commitment either, just a few minutes every day to change your life forever: amazing! Because of Deanna and her Block Therapy practice, I'm more health conscious and able to live a fit, healthy, positive life today. I couldn't have done that before.*

Albert Einstein said that coincidences are God's way of staying anonymous. I'm so grateful; I was struggling so much that fateful day I gave it a try. My wife is now a Block Therapist, sharing and teaching block; her injuries and daily pain have vastly improved, and we have even started a business together, combining Block Therapy and our love of golf. Amazing. " A block of wood? Are you kidding me?"

Chapter 5

Injury – A Different Approach

One day, while working on myself, I had an epiphany: I saw how an injured spinal cord could be sparked back to life. It was an inspired moment. I had a cozy little house by the river, a very spiritual place where my self-work really came to life. I would light candles, put on music, and sink into my tissue, losing myself in the sensations and realizations that would surface. And now, like a flash, I saw the severed ends of a spinal cord reaching out to each other, reuniting and flowing. I came out of the meditation with a start, heart pounding, more excited than I had felt in ages.

I had a mission: find someone with such an injury and put my theory to the test.

This didn't prove as easy as I thought. I never imagined it would be so hard to find someone confined to a wheelchair who would be willing to accept my offer of unlimited free treatments until he or she could walk again. I realized later I probably sounded nuts.

That didn't stop me though, and finally, after a year of searching, I saw an article in the newspaper about a young man who had broken his neck diving into a lake. He had been in the hospital for eight months and was about to be released. I visited him and told him of my plan, and he accepted my offer. The journey began.

He was a quadriplegic. He had to be belted into his chair, and had minimal movement in his shoulders. His shoulder blades had frozen up and around his neck, probably displaying the posture he had had at the moment the force fractured his spine. Everything was jammed and hard in his neck. I had a lot of work to do.

I wanted to put significant time into this at the beginning to see what I was dealing with. I decided to take five weeks away from work and make this my focus, spending a minimum of four hours a day on him. We made rapid progress. His shoulder strength and range of motion were the first obvious changes. It really hit home when his dad came over, about three weeks into the project, and said, "Wow, it looks like he's melting". Those were my very thoughts upon seeing him that day.

His shoulders had moved back to a more correct alignment, broadening their radius and lengthening the look of his neck. The tissue was also a healthier color, pink rather than grey. It looked warmer. With that came even more range of motion and strength in the area.

This led me to do research on thermodynamics. I was always a science nerd, with a special love for physics, so having a reason to study thermodynamics wasn't a stretch. As I read, I was thrilled to see that these laws helped to explain why I was getting the results I was. The second law really caught my attention: "Nature abhors a gradient".

This basically means that where there is a gap nature is going to fill it in. I meditated on it, applying it to my patient. I imagined the force that torqued his neck, causing enough damage to break it, and the response of his body in that moment.

I was already aware that the traditional way of dealing with acute injury was limiting. I was never fond of icing, and intuitively took a different approach, one contrary to what I had learned in university. There they taught us that for the first forty-eight to seventy-two hours you should limit inflammation to the site of injury to prevent further damage.

I am not formally religious, but I believe in God and a divine pattern, and this has guided me from the beginning. In that context, it didn't make sense that the body's first response to injury is inflammation, yet we are taught to suppress it. Why would the body naturally respond in this way to stress if it weren't meant to help?

The first person besides myself on whom I tested my theory was my mother. She was golfing one day, phoned me from the course, and said she had sprained her ankle. She came to see me immediately. It was indeed a bad sprain. My schooling had taught me to apply the RICE method: Rest, Ice, Compression and Elevation; but I had something different in mind.

She was in a lot of pain, so I started gently. I had been doing this work long enough that I put my trust and faith completely in my hands. If I were doing something harmful, my hands wouldn't be guided to do it.

As I applied gentle consistent pressure to her ankle, she began to calm down. I instructed her to breathe deeply and settle in. Knowing that pressure overrides pain, I knew that if she could get into a consistent breathing rhythm, the sensation would be positive. Sure enough, before long I was applying more pressure and the ankle was looking better.

I spent thirty minutes on the site of injury, the ankle and calf, and then asked her to stand. I held her hand as she walked around and she definitely was much better than she had been when she had walked in. I showed her what to do that night and said I would come to her house in the morning.

When I came over the next day she had a big smile. She let me know in no uncertain terms that she had experienced a lot of pain the night before, but that now she felt about seventy percent better. The swelling had decreased significantly and she had better range of motion. I went all in that morning; and that proved to be the last treatment she needed for what had likely been a severe second-degree ankle sprain.

So as I reflected upon my patient's spinal fracture, I realized that it was essentially like a sprained ankle. Only the amount of force that had gone in and the structures involved were different.

The fact that there was a break in the system was what mattered, and how it was handled from there would determine the result.

I could imagine that once a force enters the body, the brain goes into "fix" mode and sends blood to the site, filled with all the requirements for repair. But as in a massive car accident, help is required.

Imagine a ten-car pile-up on a highway. People are injured, debris is everywhere, and fire trucks, police cars and ambulances are sent to the rescue. These trucks require manpower, gasoline to get them there, and all sorts of support to ensure that they can save people's lives and clean up the mess so traffic can resume. But imagine this happening on an isolated road, with no help at hand, and a freeze setting in. It will take a lot longer for flow to resume and people will likely die.

This last scenario describes what happens in injuries where we apply the RICE method. There has been some kind of crash, cells are in danger, there is debris everywhere, and help is required. Freezing the area and stopping inflammation is the last thing we should be doing. Blood carries the ingredients necessary to rebuild whatever tissue has been affected: skin, muscle, tendon, ligament, bone . . . The body knows how to fix itself; it just needs the right assistance. We can trust that if something has been damaged, inflammation is bringing materials to repair it.

It's like baking a cake.

When we bake, the raw ingredients are eggs, flour, sugar and butter. Combined, they are still simply batter. It is leaving them in the oven that turns them into something delicious. Similarly, when the body inflames an injured or stressed site, it is sending the raw ingredients to rebuild that specific tissue; our task is to heat the area appropriately so as to catalyze the process.

If you freeze batter, it is frozen batter. If you bake it, it becomes cake. If you freeze an inflamed injury, the raw materials remain inert. Worse than that, there is still a gap in the system. Again, whether you have torn soft tissue or broken bone, it is a gradient that nature will fill in. If it isn't handled to promote repair, the gap sucks in the surrounding netting, or fascia, creating scar tissue. This changes cellular alignment -- one of the principal factors in aging.

Heat, then, is needed to bake tissue. With my technique, heat is generated by direct pressure combined with proper diaphragmatic breathing. Proper breathing is truly the missing link when it comes to health and beauty. Let me explain how it heats up the body.

When the diaphragm muscle is working, it moves up and down in the core. It is floor to the heart and lungs and ceiling to the abdominal organs. If it is functioning properly, it is in continual motion, performing an internal massage. This promotes optimal blood flow to all cells and keeps our tissue at the uniform temperature of 98.6 degrees Fahrenheit.

When there is collapse in the core -- and there is for everyone --this muscle isn't working to full potential. We are born using the diaphragm to breathe, but pain, fear and stress cause us reactively to hold the breath. Over time this becomes habit, and secondary muscles in the upper chest gradually take over for the diaphragm.

With no continual movement in the core, the diaphragm, the foundation of the rib cage, weakens and everything starts to cave in. Not only does the muscle decline -- it becomes compressed and misaligned, making it almost impossible to activate.

This is critical. Without proper functioning of the diaphragm, everything changes. Every state of the body -- physical, mental, emotional and spiritual -- is affected by how we breathe. The diaphragm connects us to prana, the life force. Lacking that, the body exists merely as a container for survival, rather that an evolved, conscious entity.

Using the diaphragm is like turning on the furnace in a building; breathing with the chest is like heating one room with a space heater. Or, to use another analogy: the diaphragm is like an inboard motor; the secondary muscles, the trolling motor. The diaphragm is the engine designed to feed the body with oxygen and clean the cells of waste. When it breaks down, all systems and functions suffer.

Getting back to my patient: I spent eight months diligently working to get him to walk. We made remarkable progress in that time. He gained significant function and sensation in his arms and shoulders, and could even bend forward and sideways in his chair, bringing his body back up to a seated position.

The challenge for me was that he wasn't doing the work I needed him to do. I was creating space for blood and oxygen to awaken tissue; I needed him to strengthen his body with exercise. Eventually I realized I had reached a wall and ended the treatment.

I had learned much about myself and my work -- I actually coined the term Fluid Isometrics during my time with him. I will be forever grateful for this experience.

Tammy Gibson

The day I saw that block of wood on the floor with its intriguing logo just over five years ago changed my life forever! I was at a friend's place and immediately needed to know what it was for. Within days my husband and I were meeting with Deanna Hansen, founder of Block Therapy and Fluid Isometrics, and we were introduced to the revolutionary and life changing, self-care bodywork practice called Block Therapy.

I have been a competitive amateur golfer for over 30 years, and, before I met Deanna, had been suffering with chronic right hip and shoulder pain for a number of years. My shoulder pain was due to an old baseball injury from my 20s (I was in my mid 50s when I met Deanna). There was a lot of scar tissue in there, and my mobility in my golf swing was restricted. And my hip pain was from…who knows what?…repetitive motion of the golf swing maybe?

Once I got my Block Buddy and started doing Block Therapy every day, the results were truly amazing! Within 3 weeks, the pain in both my hip and shoulder had subsided. I could feel the fascia release in those areas. My shoulder range of motion was increasing. I didn't have to cringe at the end of every golf swing, waiting for the twinge of hip pain. And some wonderful side benefits appeared: more energy, better digestion and elimination, 8 pounds lost in three weeks, and I generally felt better overall! All due to Block Therapy.

Block Therapy is a unique bodywork practice that does what no other therapy out there does. It is able to release fascia at the deepest level, bringing life and function back to tissue that was compressed, scarred, and causing me pain. The thing I like best about it is that I can do it myself, at home, on my own time. It is so easy!

The results for my health and my golf game were awesome. Not only did I get rid of my pain and increase the range of motion in my swing; I gained 15 yards off the tee! I think that's pretty amazing for a woman in her mid 50s!

My husband Barry (who is a Golf Professional) and I knew that this was something special. We were so impressed with Block Therapy that we teamed up with Deanna and created a Block fore Golf program. I also knew I wanted to share this with others, so I took the training and became a Certified Block Therapy Instructor.

My husband and I have now started a business together, integrating Block Therapy with golf swing body assessments, providing golfers and athletes with a unique program that can get to those problem areas that other fitness and performance programs are unable to address.

Block Therapy is MUST DO for your health and well-being, both body and mind, and we thank Deanna for bringing this to us and the world!

Chapter 6

Aging Has a Pattern

In 2006, a therapist who had heard about the results I was getting reached out to me. She had been seeing a patient with chronic back pain regularly for years, but had only been able to provide temporary relief. After a few sessions with me, the patient's symptoms vanished.

This started a new phase for me: now I needed to be able to explain what I was doing and why. It was a challenge, because I hadn't developed this technique rationally -- it had simply happened. The running joke in the beginning was, every time the therapist would ask me why I did something, I would say "Just go with the flow". That wasn't the response she wanted.

This pushed me to further my research. I had to make logical sense of something that to me was magical. Logic and magic don't usually sit in the same room.

I had never been an avid reader, but that changed. I was searching to make sense of what I had uncovered. I had noticed that although my hands moved in a seemingly random way when working in tissue, there was in fact an order to the pattern.

I was at that time reading The Ancient Secrets of the Flower of Life[1], and was learning about the Fibonacci sequence and the Golden Mean Spiral. With mounting excitement, I realized that this was the very pattern my hands were following.

The Fibonacci sequence is a progressive series of numbers that proves to be the mathematical foundation of everything in nature. For those who read The Da Vinci Code[2], it was the secret discovered on the back of Leonardo Da Vinci's painting, "Vitruvian Man". The sequence is 0+1=1, 1+1=2, 1+2=3, 2+3=5, 3+5=8, 5+8=13, . . . This is the measured basis of a spiral pattern recurrent in nature and epitomized by the nautilus seashell. It is the architecture of creation. The Golden Mean Spiral is the energy that runs through the building blocks of time.

Observing my hands at work, I saw that they were spiraling into dense layers of tissue. I had taken Cranial Sacral Therapy years before and learned about the "Energy Cysts" that steal the prana, the life force, from the body. I began to see in my mind what my hands were seeing.

I had the privilege of living beside a river. I noticed eddies created at the banks wherever there was an obstruction to flow.

---

1   Drunvalo Melchizedek, The Ancient Secrets of the Flower of Life (1998)
2   Dan Brown, The Da Vinci Code (2003)

I had learned through my studies that everything in nature is a reflection of the whole. I trusted that all I was seeing and feeling was connected and began to make greater sense of this work and its results.

It became apparent that if everything created conforms to this pattern of numbers, so too must the tissue as it migrates toward the earth through time. It would help if we could watch our cellular flow speeded up over years, but that isn't possible. What I could see was that wherever there was obstruction in tissue, my hands naturally followed the spiral pattern to release the tension.

Again I wish to emphasize: I didn't think this up. Over years I intuitively allowed my hands to move in the tissue, not purposefully guiding their direction, but following the path of least resistance. When I would consciously observe what they were doing, I could not discern any pattern.

Here is the best visual analogy I can offer to explain the principle. Imagine smoke leaving a pipe. Closest to the source of heat, the smoke makes a wavelike pattern. As it moves farther away, it begins to spiral until finally the threads appear chaotic. I live on the thirteenth floor of my building and can see smoke stacks in the distance; the same pattern is visible. I connected that phenomenon to what I was sensing with my hands and realized that this is exactly what happens to our cellular alignment as we age. And so what my hands were doing was tapping into the very seams of time and unlocking them.

I knew that this was the case because my own body had gone through an incredible transformation. I was becoming "younger". All of the accumulated effects of time and physical neglect were disappearing and I could feel that my body had awakened.

In university, I learned the word "necrotic", referring to dead tissue in the body. That never made sense to me. How could there be "dead" tissue in a living body? I have come to understand that there isn't: only tissue in hibernation.

This puts a different spin on aging. If tissue can be reawakened, then aging is only a function of compression. If tissue can decompress and resume flow, then aging as we know it is dead!

Myrna Irwin

Block Therapy is the best thing I have EVER done for my body! I took the introductory classes with the intention of lowering my stress, plus it was something I could do to keep my body as healthy as possible as I age. Results were pretty much immediate for the stress, and, as I continue the practice, many amazing transformations have been happening.

The first thing I noticed was that the essential tremor in my head was gone; next, the rosacea on my face was gone; and later, the psoriasis on my arms cleared up. Then an amazing thing happened on a day that I had just completed the lower body class. That evening

I was removing a pan from the oven when I accidentally spilled hot grease on my leg, over the knee. It immediately bubbled up and was so very painful. I put a loose gauze pad over it when I went to bed that night. When I woke up in the morning it was just a dry crust, no pain or redness whatsoever. I have never seen anything heal as fast as that.

A year before I started Blocking I had a tear in my meniscus that still bothered me, and I couldn't bend that knee much or kneel on it. I have to say that knee is as good as new now!

Deanna has literally and figuratively 'opened' my eyes. The heavy, puffy lids are gone; my eyes are more open, and I now have the tool and the ability to keep them that way. My hair is thicker and healthier. I feel good in this 73 year old body.

A really wild healing has occurred in my stretch marks. I got a healing crisis rash on each side of my abdomen, and when the rash healed the stretch marks were gone! Still have stretch marks surrounding those areas, but I am totally impressed with what Blocking can do.

Overall, my posture has improved, my feet are aligning, and it just feels so great to be in control of my health and wellbeing. I don't plan ever again to go to my doctor with aches and complaints and hear the YAGO diagnosis (You Are Getting Old).

Both the BT instructors and the BT Members are a huge inspiration with their helpful information and the amazing health improvements they write about. I especially love hearing from people who have had years of pain or stiffness or migraines, along with the years of expensive medications and hours in doctors' offices, who are finally getting relief with the Block and their very own breath. It's a beautiful combination.

Thank you Deanna for caring enough to bring the Block to life to give life to our cells and a healthier life to us all!!! Breathe and Believe

Chapter 7

Cellular Migration

I started my journey of discovery in my abdomen. That is where my hand dove instinctively into the tissue; that is where I began exploring an entirely new reality. As I worked to soften my tissue and strengthen my breathing, everything changed. The work with my hands was creating the space to expand my breath. I recognized that the crucial point was the exhalation. I used that internal action to build resistance around my hand as it dove into the pain. Not resistance that would forcefully restrict my breath; but enough to take control of the sensation and release it when I exhaled.

I learned to use this whenever I was feeling pain, stress or fear. It created movement as opposed to my being frozen with fear. The movement arises from the melting of frozen fats, which releases tension that binds tissue in compression. It took years of personal transformation, and the examples of hundreds of others who turned the furnaces back on in their bodies, for me to understand what was happening, assisted by my study of the laws of thermodynamics.

In Healing Ancient Wounds, The Renegades Wisdom[3], it states that the fascia can seal and bind with a force up to 2000 pounds per square inch. I have no doubt that this is true, having spent thousands of hours connecting to and melting through my own and others' tissue. Here is where we get down to the basis of how the magic works.

Magnets are attracted to, or repelled from, each other, depending on their polarity. Positively and negatively charged magnets will reach out to each other and pull together, like lovers in an embrace. As with teen love, those bonds can be overwhelming and if they aren't healthy, it may be necessary to put some space between the lovers. Unless the love is pure, distance will usually calm the attraction.

Every cell has its home: a place where it resides in perfect alignment with every other cell. Through conscious breathing we energize our cell walls enabling them to maintain their shape and position. The perfectly aligned cell has a balanced distribution of positive and negative ions, with the optimal amount of space; this makes it buoyant, like the balloon filled with air. Now imagine how you sit at a desk in front of your computer. Notice how you collapse in a forward rotational direction. When you are sitting slouched in

---

3   John F. Barnes , Healing Ancient Wounds, The Renegades Wisdom (2000)

your chair, your rib cage and pelvis are closer together. Try it. Put your hand on your rib cage and slouch. Where does it go?

The rib cage falls into the core, squishing everything. This wasn't always the normal posture of the individual. For a standard of comparison, it is worth viewing films from earlier decades. My Dad loved watching old movies; the American Movie Channel was his favorite station. Countless times I would sit with him while a movie from the forties was playing. I was always amazed by the posture of the women. They had such beautiful shoulder to hip ratios, no matter their size. It was their posture and how it held their shape that made them all so appealing. Their cells were positioned where they should be -- they hadn't migrated too far from their natural resting place.

One of the biggest health challenges we face today is technology. For all the gifts it brings, it promotes age-accumulating posture as well as well as generating frequencies that are damaging to cells. I am especially concerned for today's youth. Their posture has deteriorated far more rapidly than that of previous generations. They are constantly bending forward, focusing on screens with minute writing, turning their world into one where most of their time is spent in their heads. We have forgotten how to balance body, mind and spirit -- how to be healthy human beings.

Breathing is the most important aspect of health. Breathing properly with the diaphragm muscle, every moment, is the only

Breathe Life Into Your Fascia

way to ensure optimal oxygenation and detoxification to each and every cell. It is what our bodies are designed to do. But because our alignment is off balance from years of unconscious living, we are going to have to work to get this muscle functioning properly.

We have all been told at one time or another to sit up straight. Slouching doesn't look good. It makes people appear less present -- and that is exactly the problem. To be conscious of posture we have to be living in the moment, applying awareness at all times to how we position ourselves in the world. Sounds like a lot of work, but in Yoga it is termed "effortless effort". Anything worthwhile requires effort, and if you look around you can see that more and more people are putting tons of effort into having the body and health they desire. Like me -- before my discovery I put a great deal of time, energy and money into trying to look and feel better. As I have said, it didn't work, and, in fact, took me to a less healthy place.

The Yogic way is "effortless" because of the magnetics. When we are perfectly aligned and consciously breathing, we are inflating our cells to make them light and buoyant. This counteracts gravity's pull. The result: a body with ease of movement, healthy youthful cells, and the space to create a beautiful life with purpose and passion.

First, we need to understand alignment. We are like a building. The foundation and structure determine the stability and safety of those within. Again, it all comes down to how we breathe. The diaphragm needs sufficient room in the core to move up and down and keep the cellular residents clean and fed. If the rib cage, pelvis, shoulder girdle and neck are not aligned, it affects the shape of the core and inhibits the functioning of this all-important muscle.

Look at a healthy baby: its belly rises and falls with each breath. A baby isn't walking yet, so gravity hasn't accumulated in its tissue.

The single most important influence on our development over time is gravity. Gravity exerts a continual drag on our cells, and does so relentlessly. It has the greatest impact on objects that are dense. A conscious diaphragmatic breather has cells that are like a balloon containing the perfect amount of air to enable it to defy gravity, floating lightly, effortlessly. When we aren't breathing properly, our cells are like deflated balloons, sinking to the earth. Lack of air increases the density of a balloon; the same applies to us. Only when we position our bodies correctly will they have room to breathe.

The posture of the younger generations now is markedly different: older. It isn't uncommon to see a teenage girl with a Dowager's hump, or a tall, slender girl with a muffin top. These are indicators that the foundations in the body are not being acknowledged and the structure is collapsing. Cells are migrating away from their natural resting place, causing the walls to become thin and weak.

Consider how much the world has changed in the last twenty years. The current generation of twenty-year-olds grew up in front of the computer. The forward focus demanded of technology has accelerated their aging process. Their internal space has been drastically reduced by the collapse of the rib cage into the core, which stopped them from breathing with the diaphragm, causing a deflation and resultant compression of the cells, which in turn has made their bodies hard and dense and more susceptible to the force of gravity. In essence, their cells are running away from home (migrating) at a younger age and with greater speed.

Perfect alignment means every single one of your 100 trillion cells is sitting exactly where they should. A perfectly aligned body has optimal space. Good health requires space for blood to bring life and take away waste. Without space the body becomes malnourished and dirty: acidic. This deflated, toxic system not only has cells that have migrated away from their natural resting place; these cells are also getting squished together, forming unhealthy bonds. This body also has more waste running through it, leaving a residue that is literally gluing to itself. This combination of collapse and toxic residue has bred a perfect storm. The good news is that it can be diverted.

Janice Watson

We were introduced to Block Therapy while I was looking for an alternative treatment for my 14 year old daughter who has scoliosis.

Specialists told us that she would have to wear a back brace for 9 – 12 months during her growth spurt. The thought of her having to wear a thick mold around her mid section was unbearable, so we decided to pursue block therapy.

Since then my daughter does block every day, and throughout this time the specialist has been monitoring her and has been amazed at her progress! Her posture has improved and she has minimal pain in her back and she is moving so freely. She plays competitive sports, and without the block she would be in a lot of pain. Her goal is to continue blocking while improving her posture, and to be an educator for the younger generation. Thank you Block Therapy!

Jordyn – age 14

Block Therapy has helped me in so many ways and I really think it is something that every person should do. For me, Block Therapy has really helped with my scoliosis. My back was always really sore and it got to the point where I would need to wear a brace. It was so uncomfortable and my mom and I knew that this wasn't going to work so we started Block Therapy and since then my muscles in my back feel so much looser and I rarely have any pain. My scoliosis didn't get worse (which is a good thing) and now my curve isn't as pronounced in my lower back (have an S shaped curve). Block Therapy helps with my sore muscles, and as an elite athlete I put them through a lot. When my muscles get sore I block and it does the trick as they feel softer and looser. Block Therapy makes you aware of your breathing and your posture and I think that everyone should give it a try!

Taylor – age 10

I love Block Therapy because it has made me feel so much better and whenever I am stressed I go on the block and it gets all the bad thoughts off my mind. One night after my dance I started to feel something in my throat and it made me uncomfortable and then I started crying and my mom tried to calm me down. In the end we went to Deanna's and she sat down and I sat on her lap and she just massaged my chest and neck and after I was done it felt so much better. After that I thought that she was amazing and that's why I LOVE BLOCK THERAPY!

Ben – age 8

I like to see Deanna and Quinn because they are funny and nice and I like how they make me do Block Therapy. When I am anxious, I breathe through my tummy and it makes me feel better and calm. Blocking makes my tummy feel loose and other things like my feet. I love Block Therapy. If I didn't have it, whew, would I ever be tight!

Chapter 8

What You Think You Become

It is worth repeating: the unhealthy bonds resulting from compression seal with a magnetic force of up to two thousands pounds per square inch. Think of all that pressure and what it would do to a cell. I strongly encourage you to watch David Bolinsky's video The Life of a Cell[4], understanding that this video is about the perfectly balanced cell. To this day when I watch it, it brings tears to my eyes. Each of our hundred trillion cells is a universe, with infinite interactions perpetually occurring within its walls. It gives a whole new perspective on life, and shows how we need to treat our cells with love.

We take our bodies for granted, and then complain when they don't do what we expect them to. We curse at the chronic pain; we hate the ballooning belly. Believe me, I know. I lived it for years.

---

4 David Bolinsky, The Inner Life of a Cell (2010)

Nothing in my life took precedence over the stress I felt about my belly. It was hard, round, big, and full of shit. It made me feel ugly. Reading The Celestine Prophecy[5] was my turning point. When I learned that "what you think, you become", the realization of what I was doing to myself hit me like a freight train. I had been suffering for years because I hated myself. It wasn't because I was worth hating; it was because I hated. This was a huge breakthrough for me. I changed a thought pattern and that eventually changed everything.

I learned that thoughts have frequencies that emanate as waves. The frequency of HATE is very different from that of LOVE. Gregg Braden's book Walking between the Worlds, the Science of Compassion[6], taught me that the frequency of love is the same as the frequency of healthy DNA. This makes perfect sense: love and health have the same resonance. Fear has a much slower frequency than love, and lower cellular vibration; Braden states that the codons in the DNA shut down when fear passes through tissue.

Fear is a long slow wavelength and activates very few of our DNA antenna's.

Love is a short, fast wavelength, which activates many more antennas.

I put a lot of thought into this concept, and how it might bear upon the appearance of cells.

---

[5] James Redfield , The Celestine Prophecy (1993)
[6] Gregg Braden, Walking between the Worlds, the Science of Compassion(1997)

Masara Emoto has done beautiful research that shows the shapes water droplets assume in response to different sounds. For example, heavy metal music creates an asymmetrical, stressed-looking pattern whereas Beethoven's Pastoral[7] creates a harmonious, symmetrical one.

This is a beautiful demonstration of what the eye can't ordinarily see: that when we send hateful thoughts to others or ourselves, our cells take on that ugliness, which strengthens with time and gravity.

It is helpful to connect these very significant points to our understanding of magnetics in tissue. If negative thinking causes the codons in the DNA to shut down, it adds to the compression already underway. You can feel the charge in a room filled with excitement, as at a concert, as compared to the charge in a room where there is conflict and chaos. When we feel attacked, we reactively pull away and hold our breath, setting up a shield of tension to ward off the incoming frequency.

A neutral, balanced charge is the ideal to strive for. It allows room to travel on either side of the line. Loving, peaceful thoughts based in compassion and forgiveness create a like cellular expression. This is healthy! Unfortunately, most of us are stuck in thoughts of fear and stress, generating a magnetic charge so cells are either attracted to or repelled by each other. The ones that are attracted bind, and seal, entangled in a vortex called an energy cyst.

---

[7]   Ludwig van Beethoven, The Symphony No. 6 in F major, Op. 68, also known as the Pastoral Symphony (1808)

To achieve balance and inner peace, we must release those magnetic seals and breathe space and life back into our tissue. Cells need to be inflated so they can receive blood filled with nutrients and send away blood filled with waste. I realized years ago that this was happening to my tissue, as I would feel previously blocked areas re-awakening.

Change took many forms for me: improved vision, younger, cleaner looking skin, thicker, blonder hair, increased strength and range of motion, diminished pain . . . There really wasn't an area of my life that wasn't benefitting from the work. Even better, the patients I was working with were also receiving these transformational benefits.

With mounting excitement, I imagined a world where everyone would understand this concept. To have a simple process that everyone could realize in himself or herself would mean a world filled with happy, productive and confident people. Realizing how much change I had personally undergone, I felt I should teach this to the masses.

Karen Whyte

It was around 15 years ago. I was overweight, miserable, lost, and had no idea how I was going to get out of the hell I called my life at that time. I was using alcohol to numb myself, partying way too much, just barely existing, and hitting waves that were crashing like a bad car accident on the daily.

My boyfriend's mom gave me this book by Deanna and it involved mirror work, using your hands to heal. At the time it was too much for me as I was terrified to truly see myself in a mirror and deal with all the baggage that was so well buried deep within me. So I put away the book but hoped that one day, when I was ready, I would find it and start my healing journey.

Well, I moved a few times, and whenever I would find the book I truly felt a calling to open it . . . but had complete doubt and fear and felt utterly discouraged and that I was a complete failure in life and would never commit to anything like that . . . LIKE EVER. So I finally succumbed to my then misery and discarded her book as I felt and reconfirmed in my soul that I could never be ready to delve into all my garbage of abuse and self fulfilling prophesies; I would never be good enough to follow through on healing myself!!

After all that and making that decision . . . with another move I felt I was finally ready because I was done with making the same mistakes over and over and over, but I had forgotten I had thrown away this amazing book. I went on a rampage searching and searching for this ALL HEALING BOOK!!! I always felt such a DRAW to Deanna. I knew in my heart, her heart was a good one. I felt we in some way were the same, and I hoped I would find her again. Well, as you know, I had thrown it out, so I put it out to the Universe, if we were meant to connect and if she was meant to be on my healing path, that, somehow, it would happen.

Breathe Life Into Your Fascia

So, one day, skimming through Facebook, I saw that a friend was going to this Block Therapy session in the park nearby, and I was really wanting to find a hobby, something that I would feel connected to and passionate about. I had had quite a few drinks the night before and was super hung over all day and felt like shit, and REALLY was not in the mood, but I forced myself to go to this Block Therapy session at the park here in Morden, Manitoba.

A man named Garnie Ross taught the class. He shared that the creator of all this was Deanna. I couldn't believe my ears. It felt like it was kismet. I was meant to be here. We spent at least 90 minutes breathing and blocking and man did that block hit some sore spots!! And after the whole treatment, I got off the block, stood up . . . and felt absolutely incredible!!!

I remember getting into the car, and having to change my mirrors because I was more than two inches longer in my upper body!!! It was incredible . . . the peace, the relaxation . . . it was as though I was in someone else's body and this person felt free, and calm, and pain free for the first time in decades!!! I just knew then and there that this was a game changer.

I finally found what I had been searching for since I was a teenager training for figure skating. And as of now, whenever I am not blocking, I'm planning out the next time I will. I am unwinding my body and creating health not only on a physical level, but emotionally. I love myself more, accept myself more, and am more at peace than I ever thought was possible. I could never ever fully express the gratitude, and love I have for this amazing woman who has made it her life mission to help us all. I am officially a blocker for life Deanna!!! Bless your heart and thank you from the bottom of mine.

Chapter 9

Building Foundations

In the Yoga Teacher Training program we learned about the Yoga Sutras. To me this was like reading the bible: a way to commune with God. There are eight limbs to the sutras, only one of them being the postures, or asanas. Those who do yoga for exercise alone are probably not versed in the philosophy behind it, but I dove right into it, as it was helping me on my path to peace.

The seventh limb, the one prior to communing with God, is called Dhyana (pronounced the same as my name), which means "meditation." As I began practicing Fluid Isometrics on myself, it was exactly that for me: an accessible meditation that brought me to a place of stillness. In that stillness the understanding of Fluid Isometrics came to me. It only made sense to call it Dhyana Massage. Unfortunately, what was meant to be clever became confusing -- people started to spell my name wrong and even pronounce it incorrectly.

As I have mentioned, it was when I was working on the young man who had broken his neck that the name "Fluid Isometrics" was born.

My patient weighed two hundred and twenty pounds and was quadriplegic. It is amazing how heavy the human body is when it can't lift itself. Determined to prove my theory, I drove myself hard. I learned a lot from that experience, including my own limits. The challenge of accomplishing the impossible -- getting him to walk -- kept me going relentlessly. I finally had to stop when I could hardly lift my arm because of the pain.

This was one of the most profound learning experiences of my life. Not only did I experience with him the melting of his tissue, and connect that intuitively to what I was learning about thermodynamics; I found the perfect name for what I was doing.

It happened in a flash. I had discovered a particularly effective way to access his shoulder joints so as to melt and strengthen them. I had him on my massage table and was straddling him. I was positioned on his thighs and had his wrists in my hands. I would lean back to lift his torso off the table, and hang onto him for 15 minutes at a time. I was able to attain a position with my body that could support his weight, allowing him to hang. I really began to understand where my strength came from. It was not my arms and hands that had the power to sustain that exercise for such a long period of time; it was my core and my breath.

I was working my body differently from the way I had before, to achieve a more efficient result. This situation was unique. For one thing, he was not limited by pain. Where pain will generally determine how much of anything one can endure, it was not an issue here. The challenge was that the injury was as deep as it could be: at the spine, the center. There were many layers to melt through, and his body had been frozen in its reactive position for eight months.

This new way of positioning myself generated a lot of heat in his body. I was able to balance our energies enough to maintain the isometric contraction for a significant length of time. The cool thing about it was that as there was no alternation in the length of the muscle fibers during this time. Normally they shorten with concentric contractions and lengthen with eccentric ones. The typical bicep curl, for instance, is concentric as you bend the elbow, and eccentric as you straighten the arm. There was no such change in either his or my muscle length; rather there was one continuous, flowing movement. As this dawned on me, the phrase "Fluid Isometrics" sprang into my consciousness.

That was a great day also because on it I became aware of the significance of rooting.

Rooting is the term used to describe the action of squeezing the anus. About ten minutes into the exercise my body started to give. I was making incredible headway with melting the shoulder joints and sending blood and oxygen to the tissue, and didn't want to stop. For some reason, I instinctively contracted my anus.

Immediately I felt a surge of power that enabled me to maintain that position for another five minutes. This was something I had never experienced before.

Thus began a new postural habit. I have always been my own test subject. Something makes sense, and I become obsessive about integrating it. Fortunately I had help in this case from my yoga instructor in determining what else was necessary to provide proper pelvic alignment.

People's standing and sitting posture is a major factor in chronic joint pain and issues with aging. If we don't maintain proper foundations, tissue collapses to create false walls and floors. As I have mentioned, these block blood and oxygen flow and are the root of pain, aging and disease.

Observe the average person standing: the feet are splayed out past the hip joints. In proper alignment, the feet would be almost together and both pointing forward. One thing I have noticed is that people tend to hyper-extend their knee joints when standing -- their knees bend in the wrong direction. For a life without arthritis, chronic back pain, sexual dysfunction and constipation . . . we need to keep our cells in correct alignment, through proper posture and breathing.

When I was teaching patients to root, I would have them squeeze a book between the thighs, slightly bend the knees, align the feet and contract the anus. I learned over the years that squeezing the thighs is essential; if this action is lacking or weak, tucking the pelvis would be like a like a dog tucking its tail under -- not the goal.

It was my yoga teacher who pointed this out in my own posture. Since then I have made a point of emphasizing that action as crucial. There must be a balancing of actions if we are to align properly.

Arthritis occurs as a result of body joints rubbing together causing inflammation and eventual wearing away of cartilage. If you are properly aligned and maintain your internal space, the joints are a sufficient distance away from each other not to be in direct contact. It is when you hyperextend the knees and fall into your joint space that you create a jamming in the area. All movement from this compressed space then causes the cartilage to wear and break down. This can eventually necessitate joint replacement.

Fortunately, the body does have the ability to grow back tissue, if given what it needs. By releasing the magnetic grip of the fascia -- all the way to the bone, focusing on conscious diaphragmatic breathing and correcting posture -- you give your body the space to send healing nutrients to damaged tissue for repair.

The first time I proved this theory was with a patient I saw who had a knee replacement scheduled. He had heard about my success and in the hopes of precluding the operation, trusted the process. After 2 months of treatments and prescribed self-care work, he was able to cancel the surgery. He shared when he called that the Doctor wasn't too happy and didn't understand his decision, but to this day he has no pain in his knee and continues to maintain an active and healthy life.

How people sit also affects health. In fact, today, people say sitting is the new smoking. The average person sits far more now than in past. Pelvic compression from unconscious sitting hurts the entire body -- slouching literally crushes life from cells.

Once again, it all comes down to magnetics. When cells are supported with correct posture and breathing, the actions really don't matter. What matters is that we are conscious. Unfortunately, the average person who is sitting is involved in tasks -- often in front of the computer. When you are solely intellectually focused, you are disconnected from your body. What is essential to long-term health is conscious attention to alignment and breath.

If you sit at your job unconsciously for 8 hours a day, imagine what is happening to your pelvis. It is getting squished. Inside the pelvis are the hip joints, the organs of reproduction and elimination, and all the other structures that work together to keep us healthy and alive. They also require attention.

If people only knew what unconscious posture causes, they would take measures to create change. For example, think of the money spent on medications for sexual health.

40% of men over 40 suffer from erectile dysfunction. This really is no surprise. Erections require space for the blood to flow. Sitting unconsciously for years takes away the space in the tissue. So how can an erection occur when the roadways have become blocked through compression? It can't. But the good news is that you can reverse the symptom through releasing the magnetic seal of the fascia created over time and becoming conscious of your posture and breath.

The same is true for women, and there are even more challenges because we have a greater Q-angle -- a woman's pelvis is wider than a man's for the purpose of childbirth. On the one hand, this is an incredible gift. On the other hand, it means there is more room to "fall into" our internal space resulting in many potential issues.

How many women suffer from a weak bladder, a fallen uterus, painful periods, frustrating menopausal symptoms, endometriosis . . . the list goes on. When you are squishing your pelvis from unconscious sitting, you are pushing the organs down to the base and, for some, they even protrude from the body.

Endometriosis can be extremely debilitating. The purpose of a period is to release from the body the tissue that wasn't required to grow a baby. Every month you should be starting from neutral -- a clean slate. However, if you are unconscious of posture and breathing, the body isn't aligned to fully release all the tissue. This is also why cramping occurs at this time. If the body can't easily release the tissue as it's meant to, contractions help to force the tissue out.

Over years this unreleased tissue builds up and becomes entangled inside the pelvis. This is what endometriosis is -- when the tissue that makes up the uterine lining (the lining of the womb) is present on other organs inside your body. Fortunately, the same holds true for women as it does for men -- release the compression, breathe life into the new space, and become conscious of how you sit and stand.

Edna Guzman

My Journey to Health and Compassion

A path of reconciliation, understanding, caring and forgiveness: that would be the best way to describe my healing journey with my Block Buddy.

It all started when I was only 12 years old. My parents noticed how one of my shoulders was higher than the other. The diagnosis was easily reached after x-rays: Scoliosis. In my case, the treatments involved monthly visits to the Chiropractor for spine adjustment and sometimes weekly visits depending on the how my back behaved.

As I was an overweight girl, my self-esteem was not at its best. I learned to dress accordingly, trying not to show too much of the deviation, not realizing how my posture was making it worse. My self-image prevented me from standing tall, as I found myself at a disadvantage compared to the other girls my age.

Losing weight was a priority for me since I desperately needed to feel more attractive to others. As I grew older, my internal battle grew. I learned to manage the discomfort, pain and inflammation as it came. It was more of a denial than an acceptance, as I tried desperately to show myself and others how I could be successful in other areas of my life despite my back issues.

The real challenge came during 2016 when my back was at its worst. At age 53, pain and inflammation were increasing as I was at the peak of my career as a Training and Development Coach: a job I truly have passion for, but it required long periods of standing for hours while teaching corporate workshops.

I started meditation and Yoga to manage the pain. Compassion started to flow as I spoke to my Scoliosis realizing it had served a purpose in my life, and it was no longer needed. With a gratitude mantra, I started to search for an alternative solution. My mind and my soul knew better, despite my Chiropractor's suggestion to retire from work as my curve had reach a dangerous 30 degrees combined with disk fusion, osteoarthritis, spondylolisthesis, spine compression, and more . . .

With determination, I found Fluid Isometrics on the web. I reached out to Deanna, who explained the process and rushed the Block to my attention. At the beginning, I must confess, I thought it was a treatment to get better. I started as an obedient student, not realizing the therapy was going to change my life. I came to realize that Block Therapy is not a treatment, it is a way of life. It is about caring and listening to my body as I seek the pain and provide the oxygen and blood flow it needs. It is about connecting with myself, allowing the fascia, all the connective tissue, to be free and at peace, serving the purpose it is here to perform. The Block is my Companion, my Coach, and my Mentor through my journey to acknowledge and love the real me.

My back has straightened and the pain is gone. I lost an 8cm fibrous cyst from my uterus as it disintegrated with the Block. I am opening and maintaining space, lengthening my core while taking care of my feet. In turn and in gratitude for what the Block has done for me, I joined BTU and became the first Certified Spanish Teacher instructing others how to be whole.

I am eternally grateful for having Deanna at my side, facilitating the process with her wisdom. The Block user's community brings joy and direction to my journey. I am grateful, I am blessed.

My journey is filled with compassion.

Chapter 10

The Healing Crisis

One of the things to keep in mind when you are changing your attention and becoming more conscious is that a healing crisis may and indeed likely will occur. For a woman with endometriosis for example, there are years of built up tissue that have to be released. Once decompression begins, the body will eliminate the old accumulation. In such a case, heavy bleeding may occur at the start of the cleansing process -- a sure sign the body is doing what it needs to.

I have had many healing crises with this process over the years; in fact, I welcome them. In the moment, they teach me to be patient. Although I may be experiencing some kind of "negative"

sensation, I understand that is part of my healing. How can a body clean itself without our being aware?

A healing crisis occurs when positive energy is put into the body and negative energy is released. This is an important component of healing, as dirt and debris need to be flushed out for tissue to become healthy. The challenge is that if you don't understand it, it can be scary.

The crisis can occur in many forms: physical, emotional and mental. Physical responses can be change in pain, skin rash, mucous production, fever, diarrhea, and increased menstruation, to name a few. Emotional releases can be anger, guilt, shame or sadness. Mental releases can be old memories resurfacing, or even nightmares that reveal trapped thoughts.

What you need to understand is that anything negative that you are holding onto will present itself and be felt on the way out when an opportunity for release is granted. On the other side of the crisis, peace and calm await. The new space created by the release of old material will allow for improved flow to the cells: a must if you want to improve your cellular health.

Adhesions are really the source of your suffering. When you melt them, all the trapped waste starts to migrate out of your body. What is stuck and where it is located will determine the nature of your healing crisis.

Another challenge: it is impossible to predict how or when a healing crisis will occur. For some it can be immediate and frequent; for others it may be more drawn out. The important thing is to allow it to happen and do what you need to do to assist the process.

When cells are fed and clean, they are healthy. When they are congested and dirty, the environment is ripe for disease. In any health challenge, a healing crisis is essential.

Heather Y.

I find it a shame that we tend to be so hard on ourselves in so many ways. The Block teaches you to be kind, gentle and persuasive with your body. Love yourself, love your cells, love your new lifestyle.

My experience with Block Therapy started January 2016. I can't begin to tell you how happy I am today that I went to my first class! I was going through a very difficult time. So many negative things happened in my life, and they just kept on coming, one after the other. These things were not only happening to me, but also to people very close to me. I was feeling such a huge sense of loss, frustration and deep sadness. Trying to put on the happy face whenever I was in public was making me feel so fake, which added to my depression. I was starting to have major anxiety and panic attacks. I was feeling like everything was spiraling out of control. I was always the person people came to for guidance, and now my own world seemed to be crumbling around me . . . I was a complete mess and, sadly, I couldn't fix it.

My class time was coming up and I was preparing to bail. I debated whether I was going to go or not. How could I show up when I'd been crying all day? I decided to "put my big girl pants on" and just do it. Fake it till you make it! Who knew I was about to go through such a huge shift after only one class. That was when I knew I was hooked and I'd never go back. From feeling like an emotional train wreck only minutes before my class, I came home on cloud nine! I was so happy and excited to share my experience with my son. He couldn't believe the difference in me either. Who knew that so much emotion could be stored in your cells? Not me! But I sure know now. In fact I know so much about my body now and how it functions, how everything is connected, experiencing the mind, breath, body connection and listening to and observing what my body is "asking me" to work on . . . WOW, what an education and gift I received!

That night I purchased my block and a DVD so I could practice between classes. I started going to classes once per week and loved them. I was so happy and grateful to have found this therapy. I had other issues going on with my body due to years of improper alignment, bad posture, scar tissue and compression. There was a lot of fascia bunched up which I slowly saw melting away. One spot in particular I had had since I was a child. It is now gone. I carried that lump around for 40 years! I was also having a lot of trouble with my right leg from my hip all the way down to my foot and a bunion was starting to form. It was difficult to walk, go up and down stairs, and sleep comfortably. I no longer could do the sports and exercise classes that I loved without extreme pain. Wearing any kind of footwear was also becoming a huge challenge with the added inflammation that was occurring in my foot. Oh no! What was I going to do if I couldn't wear shoes anymore? I was given some guidance from Deanna and I started my program. The transformation was incredible! Slowly and steadily I was able to start healing these areas. The nice bonus was that it appeared that I was also losing inches here and there. I was used to slowly gaining inches. My clothes (and my shoes) started to fit better, my right thigh was no longer aching, my foot was starting to shrink back to its proper size, and my anxiety was lessening. The panic attacks stopped as well. I was starting to feel like a new me!

I had spoken to Deanna a couple of times over the phone, through texts, and also at one of her weekend intensives. She impressed me with her knowledge and genuine compassion. I knew I had found the key. This was it! This was the perfect therapy for me, and she was the person I wanted to support. Shortly after this, the Member Site was launched to the public. You can imagine that I was all over that. With this resource I was able to access so many videos that were created to target specific areas and topics. You even have the option to purchase some for your own private collection. What a gold mine!

It has been just over three years for me now. I am an avid Blocker. I block every chance I get. Usually daily, but never fewer than 4-5 times per week. I will block for 15, 30, 90, 120, even up to 180 minutes each time. I can't get enough! I find it is a great way to exercise, meditate, and self heal, and you can see results with only 15 to 30 minutes a day and one class per week. I love that I can block almost anywhere: in bed, in the car, at my desk, on the couch, in a chair, or on the floor. You can even take it with you while travelling. I have blocked on a plane and while on holiday many times. My favourite place to block is on my deck on a warm, sunny day. I find the cost minimal too. I mean, you really only need a block and some instruction. Once you get a block it will become your most precious and valued possession. With it you can become your own health care advocate. It is your magic tool that you can use anytime, almost anywhere, for as long as you want. Goodbye pills!

I continue to be blown away by the wealth of information and education I receive from Deanna and other Block Therapy Instructors. It's not just another exercise class; it's a whole community of fellow blockers coming together. How does it get any better than that?!? I am ever so grateful for discovering the benefits of Block Therapy and I can't thank Deanna enough for sharing her knowledge with the world!

Chapter 11

Another Foundation – The Power of the Tongue

Another postural action I have spent years developing is strengthening the tongue. I never really thought much about this muscle in past, except that as a kid I heard it was the strongest muscle in the body, which never made sense to me -- I couldn't lift a chair with my tongue.

Then one summer, doing yoga at the lake, I made a discovery.

I suffered at that time from chronic neck pain, which was exacerbated by my work. Leaning over a massage table always put my neck in a vulnerable position.

I had rented a cabin for two weeks, the first break I had taken in years. I was practicing forward bends on the deck, enjoying the sound of the loons, when the pain I knew so well said hello. For some reason, I contracted my tongue. To my amazement, the pain disappeared. This was noteworthy because the pain always kicked in when I bent forward. I relaxed my tongue and felt the pain; contracted it again and instantly felt relief. And so I found a new obsessive action to integrate.

I became aware of my tongue's habitual bearing: forward and to the right. I clenched the left side of my jaw more and had issues with a molar there. I realized that there is a ridge at the roof of the mouth, about a pinky nail distance from the teeth, that perfectly fits the tongue -- a docking station. Whenever I could I would move my tongue to that alignment.

This brought a whole new insight into neck pain. I had heard Dr. Oz once say that the neck weighs about ten pounds, but when incorrectly aligned can be up to a hundred pound force on the muscles of the upper back, neck and jaw. I had no trouble believing this because I personally had issues with all of those areas.

I started connect tongue alignment to vertebral alignment as so many of my patients suffered from arthritis of the neck. The forward head posture common all of us means that our vertebrae are not properly supported.

In fact, most people have such misaligned necks that there is considerable wear and tear in the joints. This is arthritis in a nutshell: inflammation of the joints due to incorrect alignment. Measures taken to remedy it will be temporary unless the neck is put back in place.

The tongue muscle is unique in that it is the only muscle in the body with just one attachment. Every other muscle has an origin and an insertion. When the tongue is properly placed, the head is repositioned and supported, maintaining proper alignment of the vertebrae. This allows the neck incredible range of motion and freedom.

This alignment is also crucial to all the structures in the area. For example, the carotid arteries, which are positioned at the front of the neck, are the main roadways supplying blood and oxygen to everything in the head: the brain, the eyes, the skin, the hair, the thyroid, the ears, etc. Using the tongue to keep the head and neck properly aligned allows optimal space for these tissues to be healthy and function with ease.

So many degenerative conditions are on the rise. One of the reasons is that we are living longer; but, in my opinion, it is the posture that is the culprit.

Dementia and Alzheimer's are a huge concern. Anyone who has taken care of a family member so afflicted knows how the experience can suck the joy out of life, not to mention creating symptoms in your own body/mind. Like everything else in the body, keeping a healthy mind requires space for the tissue. When the neck collapses in a forward, rotational direction, the brain compresses against the skull. As with the joints in the body, lack of space leads to degeneration.

We all have the ability to apply to our bodies what is necessary to maintain optimal flow so as to keep our cells properly fed and cleaned. I believe that strengthening the tongue muscle is extremely important in the prevention of mental degeneration. As with the diaphragm, if we don't focus on strengthening this muscle, the weight of the head will squish the contents in the neck, creating barriers.

The thyroid gland has many functions and is of great concern right now. There has been a 200% increase in thyroid cancer since the 1970s. Personally, I see this as a function of the effects of technology on posture. The forward head tilt from looking at screens and phones all day has dramatically changed the alignment of the average individual. There are many other factors that have made us less healthy, but compression of this organ has made it starved and dirty.

What about the eyes? Seeing is taken for granted until your vision is affected. The eyes are ball and socket joints, like the shoulders and hips. The eyeball sits in the orbit, with space between it and its container. Proper alignment of the head and neck ensures that the eyes have the space to receive nutrients, and to track in all directions.

When you look down for hours at a time, as at a computer screen, you draw your head down and your eyes move up. In fact, few people have their necks resting in a neutral position; the head is forward and down -- a function partly of the alignment of the ribcage, which we will address in the next chapter.

With this prolonged alignment, eventually the eyeballs adhere to their sockets, creating a condition similar to that of a frozen shoulder. The range of motion decreases and blood is blocked from the areas of adherence. As with other cells in the body, aging accelerates and vision is compromised. Decompressing the tissue, improving the breath and aligning the cells keep everything in the body healthy and functioning . . . for life.

Sandee Bachalo

Block therapy has changed my life. I've suffered from migraines and various types of pain as a result of car accident in my twenties. Treatments (chiropractor, massage therapy, pain medication) provided temporary relief, but I never felt I was getting better. As time went on, I was feeling foggy all the time (from ongoing pain, medication etc) and struggling to make it through the week, often collapsing on the weekend. Life was about looking after my family, work, and pain management.

Fortunately, Deanna came into my life, and for the first time I started to feel hope -- hope that I could control my pain, gain my life back, and not just try to get through the week. Participating in various intensives and having a monthly membership taught me how to use the block to continue to move my health forward and to treat my pain. I am no longer foggy. I no longer have daily pain. My use of pain medication has dramatically decreased. My migraines are greatly reduced and rare and less severe. I am constantly moving forward, releasing fascia and changing my body.

I actually feel like I am getting young . . . turning fifty shortly and I feel better than I did when I was twenty. Other people have noticed

-- *my chiropractor who has been treating me for 20 years asked me what was I doing, I was so much better and I was responding to his treatments differently (the adjustments were actually staying in place). I still see him but have greatly reduced my reliance on him and reduced my appointments by around 60%.*

Block therapy is an amazing program, capable of helping so many people. My son has used it as well, after hockey and for treating tight muscles or pain. Much better than icing it (as he was told to do when he hurt his hand recently) and taking pain medication -- he recovers quickly and never misses a game.

Thank you Deanna for bringing this to the world!

Chapter 12

Aligning the Ribcage – An Essential Component for Health

Strengthening the tongue muscle is crucial to supporting the weight of the head; but there is more to it than that. The ribcage is the foundation of the neck. Without a strong foundation, no matter how strong the tongue is, the head will be pulled forward by the collapse of the ribcage into the core.

Correct alignment and support of the ribcage is essential to the health of everything up the chain, including the shoulder joints, arms and hands, as well as the head and neck as already mentioned.

Carpal tunnel syndrome, for instance, is a common concern, especially for those on a computer all day. Surgeries and therapies are offered to provide relief, but they seldom do. Frozen shoulder is another widespread complaint -- people are told to ride it out, as there is no "cure".

These are classic cases of trying to solve a problem by attacking the symptoms while ignoring the cause. The root of all disorders of the head, neck, arms and hands is the foundation, the rib cage. If it isn't properly supported, everything else is off. The body compensates for weak foundations by collapsing to create false walls and floors. With frozen shoulder, for example, these prevent the joint from moving in its optimal range.

The ribcage affects not only what sits on top of it, but also what it squishes and compresses. When you see a picture of the organs in a textbook, you see a perfectly balanced and aligned body. But none of us is perfect, and most are far from it. Let's consider what happens to the internal organs when we collapse.

When the ribcage collapses, the entire weight of what it contains and supports --heart, lungs, thymus, shoulders, arms, head -- bears down on the abdominal space. The stomach, pancreas, liver and gallbladder get squished and displaced. Tissue compresses to provide support, blocking blood and oxygen flow.

This affects not only organ function, but also outer form. The internal space required to house the organs is depleted; as a result, tissue protrudes outward. Understanding this is essential to treating obesity.

In a balloon half full of air, if you squeeze one end, the other bulges. This is what is really going on anywhere in the body where we think we have accumulated fat. It isn't about fat; it's about displaced fascia.

It makes sense. Even in the absence of lifestyle change, we find it increasingly challenging to keep a flat belly and hourglass figure as we age. Many go to extremes to try to force the body to become what it used to be, without success. The reason is that we are approaching the issue from the wrong perspective.

The size and shape of the core is dependent on cellular alignment. It all comes back to proper posture and breathing. When the diaphragm muscle is working as it should, it continually massages the organs. Without this continual action, the organs can't do their job, and digestive and eliminatory problems arise.

We expect a lot from our bodies without considering what they need to work properly. For instance, we expect the stomach to do its job, and when it fails, we assault it with chemicals and fear. How many people take antacids and other medication to simply break down food? Then, when the food doesn't get processed and absorbed, it also doesn't get eliminated, and there is a backup of waste in the system. This attracts parasites that thrive in the acidic environment, producing their own waste and adding even more bulk. No wonder our diets don't work; what we eat only accounts for a fraction of what makes us expand.

Certainly, food is a factor. Eating fast and processed food, and too much, will unfailingly add size to the middle and the body as a whole. But this is only one piece of the puzzle. I learned from personal experience that it isn't only about calorie intake versus energy expenditure. In my twenties, when I was working hard to change my size and shape, that equation proved useless. I was eating little, exercising to the extreme -- and getting bigger. I thank God every day that I learned how to decompress. Had I kept on the way I was going, I would likely weigh three hundred pounds today.

NAFLD -- Non Alcoholic Fatty Liver Disease -- is also on the rise. This basically means that fats are trapped in the liver. Fats need a certain temperature to melt. Think of butter at room temperature compared to heating it in a frying pan. The action of working the diaphragm -- making it move up and down in the core -- creates a continual internal massage. This is like turning on the internal heating engine. Unfortunately, most people hardly use this muscle, so it weakens. Not only does this result in the collapse of the ribcage, it creates a freezing of the core, which allows fats to solidify.

The solution: turn up the heat. The challenge: the 2000 pound per square inch force sealing the body out of alignment and blocking access to this function. Fortunately, as mentioned before, I have learned how to decompress fascia, releasing this force.

What about the heart? What happens to it when the ribcage collapses? First of all, there is immense pressure on it. Imagine how you would feel if you had an elephant sitting on your chest. That is virtually what it is like for a heart enduring the weight of unconscious posture.

Along with that goes the constriction of internal space. Everything needs room to function properly; when that is diminished, stress results.

The aorta, the main artery leaving the heart, is a big tube carrying blood to feed the cells. It passes through the diaphragm before branching off to ensure that every cell is nourished. When the ribcage falls into the core, this tube gets compressed. Imagine taking a normal breath; then imagine breathing through a straw. The difference is in the amount of space available for the flow. The collapse of the ribcage takes this away, forcing the heart to work harder. It isn't that the heart is damaged or weak; it is that the space required for it to function has been diminished.

Early on I had the epiphany that scar tissue and compression were the root of all chronic physical suffering. I saw, working on myself and my patients, that as decompression occurred, tissue resumed its youthful function and appearance.

Every ailment can be traced back to cells out of alignment and deprived of space. The constant force of gravity crushes and warps us so we age and deteriorate; but we don't have to.

Rose Benjamin

Block Therapy came to me at a point when I was experiencing a ramped up and more frequent version of scoliosis pain. I couldn't travel in a car for more than 2 hours without pain, and as I stepped out of the car, I'd have to hold onto the door for a minute before walking in order to regain balance as I stabilized from the pain and stiffness. My digestion and elimination were poor and I hated looking at my puffy belly that had been with me since my teen years. My left knee hurt, especially on stairs, and a bunion on my left big toe was getting worse. I figured I'd have to get similar surgery to what I already had had on my right big toe. I felt old, as I would get out of bed in the morning and do a teetering walk to the bathroom after a poor night's sleep, often waking in pain.

I am so thankful for the invitation from a fellow natural health teacher to watch a webinar about Block Therapy. After hearing Deanna explain the process and how it affects the body, and especially after I saw how a younger person with more severe scoliosis than me had improved, I contacted Deanna about starting and experienced some hope for the first time in years. The first thing I asked, though, was, "Am I too old to start and to experience good results at age 69?" Deanna assured me and said there were older people than me doing Block Therapy.

Thus I started my journey of 3 exercises per day while I wrote about it in the 21 Day Block Blitz book that I'd had printed out. I was encouraged by an acupuncturist to see if there might be a teacher program so I could get more attention and help as I went along. After seeing the price of the program, I decided that this would be a good investment in the quality of my future. What good would it be if I stayed where I was and went on vacations, but still had to deal with the effects of a trip on the plane and pain as I moved about? Am I ever glad for that decision!

I really hadn't meant to be a teacher, but after experiencing a flatter belly, better balance, less pain, better range of motion, improved ability to remember and perform my tap dances, after just

2 rounds of the 21 day program, I decided this process had to be shared with others. As I continued, I noticed that my posture was improving, along with my ability to do yoga poses, and that I had better stamina and balance. The next year my bone density improved from an osteoporosis diagnosis I had previously been given. So many enhancements to my quality of life!

Now, as a certified teacher, after a class, I am always approached by someone who has had a breakthrough of some kind that they could not find with any other exercise. I experience such joy when I see that this natural process has affected them so profoundly! So thank you, Deanna Hansen, for all your expertise and knowledge of the body that you have shared with me and others. I am forever grateful!

Chapter 13

Introducing Block Therapy

For years, I put my professional energy and attention into patient work. This included teaching therapists my bodywork practice, Fluid Isometrics. It's interesting now to look back. Had I known what I was getting myself into, I probably wouldn't have chosen this path. But it continually unfolded before me, almost as if I had no conscious choice. By this I mean that I created things along the way in response to what others asked for, not because it was what I intended to do.

Teaching self-care was always my foremost passion. I once tried teaching individuals how to use of their own hands to decompress tissue. This did not prove viable; the fascia, with its incredibly powerful seal, would fight back, and if people had problems with their hands, they would find it too challenging to go deep enough to break through the seal. I had been able to teach myself this art; but that wasn't how others would be able to learn it.

In 2010, I started to experience significant physical exhaustion. I was working regularly on patients, then coming home and working equally on myself. I was caught in a cycle of needing to fix myself so I could help others; but my hands and body were suffering. There was a moment of clarity when I asked myself, Who would possibly listen to me? I was in pain, miserable, and had neglected my own need for peace and balance -- my passion and desire to help others had depleted me. Something had to change.

I had always loved doing yoga, but I had pushed it out of my life. As demands on me grew, I let go of practices I needed for balance. I decided to call my friend, an exceptional yoga teacher, and ask her to come and teach private classes to me.

She agreed. Every week she came and gave me a class. This became one of my favorite parts of the week -- it was truly a form of conscious resting. I could not have done it alone, my energies were so unbalanced.

Each session she would ask what I wanted, and every time I replied that I needed to be lying down. I had migrated to working on patients on the floor and was using my body very forcefully all day long, so I didn't feel inclined toward high impact postures; I just wanted to rest. Eventually this became our routine: she would walk into my apartment and I would be lying on my back, ready for her to guide me with her beautiful soothing voice.

Don't get me wrong -- restorative yoga can be very physical. The postures are held for long periods, allowing me to go thoroughly into them. This was what I loved. It gave me time to connect to my breath and isolate where in my ranges I was stuck. The stiffness I would feel after a session would give me the areas I needed to focus on with my hands, always guiding me deeper into the fascia than I would otherwise have gone.

Twists were among the most common postures we explored. They work the core like crazy, and help to squeeze out toxins. I would lie over a bolster to allow fuller access to the posture, and she would warn me just how deep this was and to be careful.

To me, it wasn't deep at all. I had spent years applying intense manual pressure to these areas, so I didn't actually feel much. I had a wooden Yoga block from my Iyengar yoga days; I said I wanted to use this instead of the soft bolster. The look on her face said she thought I was crazy, but I went ahead.

It was magic. I now had a tool that would allow deeper than ever access to my tissue. This excited me tremendously because I needed to give my hands a break, but didn't want to stop the self-work I had grown to love. I played with the block for some time, feeling the beauty of the wood and how deep it could get, far deeper than my hands, as I was using my own body weight to reach the pain. The wood seemed to communicate effortlessly with the bone.

There was just one problem.

There were areas I wanted to access that I couldn't quite reach, because there are no straight lines in tissue. The sharp edges of the block were proving painfully problematic in these places.

One of my therapists was also a woodworker, so I asked him if he could round the edges of the block to make it friendlier to areas like the armpit and groin. He would make changes, I would try the new prototype for a while, and then more changes would be made, until we finally found the right shape. Then the challenge became the wood itself.

Because the block would be in contact with the skin, I was adamant that it must be free of all toxic substances -- no lacquer, stain or glue. The wood had to be raw, and of a single solid piece. Unfortunately, wood cracks as it dries, which presented yet another set of problems. It wound up being a two-year process, but we persevered and ultimately succeeded.

For years, people told me I needed to clone myself. This proved figuratively to be the answer. A tool that is able to replace the therapist. All you need is instruction and a willingness to transform. The name of the tool: The Block Buddy. For those who practice Block Therapy -- an appropriate name -- it becomes your friend for life!

As with Fluid Isometrics, once I started using the Block Buddy on my own body, I began to use it with my patients. My initial intent was to give them a home program so they wouldn't need to see me or the other therapists as frequently. I didn't want lifelong patients; I wanted to get people to a place where they could look after themselves.

One of the biggest problems for people, as I have mentioned many times, is that they don't breathe from the right place. Even if patients only use the Block Buddy in one position that helps them maintain the habit of breathing diaphragmatically, that is of immeasurable value. Gradually, though, I started to give patients more positions to do, and it really caught on.

That inspired me to teach a class. Everything I did in the treatment room could be accomplished with the Block Buddy, using body weight and gravity to supply the force. I taught a few single classes, and people really liked them, but they said they needed more instruction. So I decided to put six guys I knew, including my boyfriend, brother-in-law, and lawyer, through the wringer. I planned six classes for them to see what would result.

Everything I do for the first time, is the first time. This is both a blessing and a curse: I have the freedom to make everything up as I go, but no reassuring framework. This is often how it feels for me. Rather than using a script or template, I listen to what people say they want and need and do my best to accommodate them.

I have to say, though, this was fun. As I was totally comfortable with everyone, the jokes were flying; at the same time, my pupils took what we were doing quite seriously. I was teaching them how to find pain on purpose, something counter-intuitive for most, and keeping them in positions for 3-5 minutes. The ones I knew well, who had been patients of mine for years, were comfortable with the work; but there was one new guy, a friend of my lawyer's, who was the polar opposite of flexible. He was moaning in pain and I felt I needed to go to him. When I asked him where it hurt, back, shoulders, hips, his response was simply: Yes!

The feedback was great. There was follow through, and it struck me that this was something I could turn into a program. I had just moved into a new clinic, and had room to hold classes for six at a time.

For the next two years I balanced patient work with teaching. As much as patient work will always be part of my life, I knew that if I wanted to get Block Therapy out into the world, I would have to make that my main focus. It was time to begin a new adventure. I closed my clinic, and for the first time in 20 years, didn't have a place to go to work.

The two years following were a rollercoaster ride. I decided to teach Block Therapy to larger groups. I rented space in a church that held up to forty people and began marketing the classes.

My nephew Quinn was eighteen. I had always felt he would be part of Fluid Isometrics, but I would never push or suggest it. He had just started Business School at university when I held my first large class. He came to it and was sold.

He told me he wanted to quit school and dive into Block Therapy. Inside I was beaming; the thought that he wanted this filled me with joy. Then he asked if I would tell his parents he wanted to quit school. That threw me: I still wasn't sure how I was going to get my message out to the world, although I did know it would require an army. We talked about it at length and I agreed to be his advocate.

Quinn had always been a natural athlete; bodybuilding was now his passion. He was like me: when he found something he loved, he would dive right in. His training at the gym had certainly enabled him to bulk up, and he had grown significantly in the last year. He also worked at a supplement store, and was consuming large amounts of its products.

I told him my opinion of these, and said that if he really wanted to help me share the benefits of Block Therapy, we needed to test his body and see what the practice alone could do for him. He agreed to stop taking supplements. Thus began a whole new path for us both. I had no interest in spending time at the gym. Thankfully, Quinn took on the task of integrating what he learned from me into his training, and it didn't take long to see remarkable changes in him.

Working on patients for years for hours a day, I had grown very strong. Fluid Isometrics is a perfect name and benefits both the patient and the therapist. The technique requires slow, continual pressure at a steady pace. That is what allows such deep access to people's tissue without undue stress. You acclimatize to pressure in the tissue when it is consistent. This requires of therapists a strong connection to their own core and breath.

So I didn't become strong in the traditional manner, and I wished to translate what I had intuited over the years into a system that could teach people how to become strong themselves. This was fun, as I would work with Quinn (already a super strong guy) and share a different approach to working out.

One night we went to the gym together to make some changes to his routine. I wanted to teach him how to strengthen his fascia, not his muscles. The act of working on people's fascia and following their tissue naturally created a pattern of movement that I adopted. I wanted to integrate that into his existing program, with some minor tweaks to the movements of lifting weights and connecting to his breath.

He was so excited. After he began to apply this, he was blown away by how much stronger he was becoming without the typical post workout pain; and the cool part is, he was using less weight. The process generated an overall cellular integration in the area of focus and created a clean and symmetrical appearance. With the decompressing component of Block Therapy, his body quickly responded. Before long, he was getting noticed.

Quinn Castelane

When I was first introduced to Block Therapy, I was interested in how it could benefit my bodybuilding career. I had tried pretty well all legal supplements, stretching, and what the media told us to do to get bigger, leaner and stronger. After a few sessions of Block Therapy, I found that my pre- and post-workout recovery was far better than any I had experienced from supplements. I could recover faster, improve the pump and blood flow in the gym, change my symmetry and proportion -- all because of targeting the fascia system. Little did I know, this practice does so much more than just benefit my workouts. It has literally changed my life in nearly every way possible. How? Because we target the fascia system and make this a lifestyle! You don't just view Block Therapy as something you do for 15 minutes per day; you integrate all aspects of Deanna's knowledge into your life.

The body can be understood as a complex system -- so complex that the average person doesn't even know where to begin in the health and healing process. Deanna takes a different approach. She helps us understand the body through analogy, in ways that all ages can understand. And not just 'understand', but take action to manage and heal ourselves.

I feel I have found and mastered the solution to living a healthy, long and enjoyable life. I can manage my pain, my alignment, even issues such as disease, because I now have a different understanding of the body. It's simple: we need to create space in the body, oxygenate our cells, and then create proper postural foundations. As long as the fascia is open and our systems can flow optimally, the body takes care of the rest. It can heal itself. This is why Block therapy is the missing link in self care.

It is not only the physical body I am referring to, but also the mental and emotional. Especially in the new millennium, anxiety, stress and depression are on the rise. Breathing diaphragmatically and literally decompressing the body so the cells can receive life, is the cure to these issues. Block Therapy can do absolute wonders for the body, and it is for everyone.

Chapter 14

Following the Flow

We are like rivers. A healthy young river has solid, narrow banks and fast, clean flow; an aging river meanders, with unstable banks and irregular flow. I live on the thirteenth floor of a high rise on the river; before this I had a house on the river. I have observed over the years what happens to flow through the seasons. As people age, they become like the aging river.

I loved my house. It was a small cabin style home -- it was like being at the lake, the way it was positioned, yet only a block away from a major city artery. The back yard was completely private and faced a park directly across the river, close to where I grew up. The view was phenomenal.

It was situated on a bend. The current flowed toward the house, at a point where the banks were wide. In the springtime the river would pound on the bank directly in front of the property, gradually undermining it. In six years of living there, we lost a significant amount of land. Meanwhile, on the other side of the river, you could see deposits causing the bank to build and extend beyond itself. At the edges, eddies would pull in debris, trapping garbage and waste.

Every year, as spring turned to summer, life would thrive on the banks. What kind of life depended on the health of the area. Where banks are healthy and flow is fast, the water is clean and wholesome life abounds. Where there are disruptions to flow and eddies are present, waste accumulates, promoting growth of algae, which attracts less savory organisms. So it is with the human body.

From my apartment, thirteen stories up, I have a different perspective -- an eagle's eye view. One spring, to the right of my building, a fallen tree had extended into the river. It was fascinating to observe how this barricade changed the current. It brought me back to the Fibonacci sequence and the way energy moves in waves and spirals.

The tree stretched quite far. It was old; its base right at the bank. It must have lost its grip with the spring flood and uprooted itself. There it sat, creating a visual display for me to study over the summer: a magnificent gift that brought clarity to my evolving insights.

Typically, foam on the surface of the water would flow in the middle, halfway between the banks. Presumably, this was where the current was strongest, the foam riding the wave like a surfer. The interesting part was what happened to the foam as it approached the area of the fallen tree.

The foam was pulled toward the tree in a spiraling pattern, accumulating on the underside. Here was a striking confirmation of everything I had been learning about the Fibonacci sequence as the underlying architecture of the universe, and the golden mean spiral as the way energy moves through it. As with the smoke leaving the pipe, I could see how the foam first traveled in a wave, then began to spiral as it moved toward the tree, and finally disintegrated into apparent chaos, where the foam was intermingling and intertwining, the threads losing any apparent order. Now I had two visuals to help me make sense of what my fingers were detecting. To stop the foam from spiraling into chaos, all that was needed was to remove the tree.

Everything in nature mirrors nature. This is loaded with meaning; among other things, it helped me put together a language with which to teach Fluid Isometrics. If you observe the movement of my hands on the surface of a body, there is no apparent pattern. This always presented a challenge when I was teaching therapists. They would ask why I did what I did, or how I knew where to go next; but the fact was that I wasn't planning the route; it was already there. The route is the path along which the tissue has sealed over time; and in that respect, as in so many others, everyone is unique. One must learn how to tap into the seams of time and let the tissue guide. This can't be explained logically. I learned to teach with visual analogy, just as nature was teaching me.

When working on patients, I could feel that under the surface chaos lay the spiral. This was where the tissue felt dense. Screwing into this density would create a release. Once the area softened, a wave of flow resumed. I loved that I could now explain the actions that my hands were intuitively taking. It wasn't chaos; the pattern was definite and followed the laws of nature.

I take the same approach in teaching Block Therapy. First I make clear that removing blocks in tissue is the single most important step to healing. This involves learning about magnetics and the two thousand pound per square inch seal. Block Therapy opens the main routes for transport and ensures that tissue temperature is conducive to optimal flow. This is why it is so effective.

We heat our tissue by a two-pronged approach: direct pressure applied with the Block Buddy, bodyweight and gravity; and proper diaphragmatic breathing. This combination is exponential in its effect. When it is maintained for an appropriate length of time, blood flow increases, feeding cells and flushing them clean. A clean, nourished environment is alkaline in nature and promotes good health. Another benefit is that adhesions between layers of fascia melt, as they are, in part, formed from solidifying fats. Combined with residue and debris, frozen fat and protein are part

Breathe Life Into Your Fascia

of the material of "The Fuzz" -- the physical manifestation of aging in tissue. Melt the fuzz, and you melt away the years.

Block Therapy does just that; and, unlike any other system, goes deep enough into tissue to attack suffering at its root: the bone. The principal challenge is that two thousand pound per square inch magnetic force, which glues the fascia to itself, and to bone. The direction of force follows the spiral pattern of energy. Like a whirlpool, it pulls in all it can grab. The fascia is gravity's root, and it spreads its tendrils over the entire physical structure, sucking itself into the internal space, displacing tissue outward, like a bulging balloon. It is called an energy cyst -- aptly named because it steals the life force.

When we apply this understanding to fitness and exercise, we see that the traditional approach doesn't make sense. In my younger years, I was the typical athlete. I played high-level volleyball, spent time doing weights in the gym, did aerobics and Tae-Bo, and tried many varieties of exercise in the moment, attempting to gain the results I wanted. The harder I worked, the worse I looked and felt.

Traditional muscle building involves holding a weight while performing repetitive contractions targeting a certain muscle or muscle group. I remember, during my first year in university, spending hours in the gym. I was bench-pressing 125 pounds, doing 100 push-ups a day, as well as working out all the other areas of my body. All I wanted was to be thin and fit. I remember walking past my Mom and her saying, "your head is too small for your body". This didn't make me happy.

Another time, again wanting to shed weight, I adopted the stair climber as my exercise of choice. I would do the highest intensity possible for 45 minutes. The front of my shirt would be soaked and I would be exhausted. I gave myself 3 weeks of this before trying on an old pair of jeans that had become snug. I was very excited; I believed they would effortlessly slide on. To my horror, they were tighter. My thighs and butt were bigger. How could this possibly be true when I was burning off tons of calories?

I get it now. All the efforts I made took away the space in my tissue for blood and oxygen flow. The struggle to attain a "hard body" resulted in a dense body. The repetitive muscular contractions and movements had shortened my tissue, making it hard and dense, not toned and sleek. This shortening also pulled my posture forward to where it had sealed with that 2000 pound per square inch force. Talk about adding insult to injury!!!

It was my practice of Iyengar Yoga that first introduced me to the concept of lengthening and strengthening. I so appreciate my years at this, as they taught me about proper alignment and energy flow. However, I was still aware that the practice alone wouldn't remove the grips sealing fascia to bone. It was only when I worked on the area of restriction that I was able to make real progress.

As I was sharing my insights with Quinn, he was awakening to the truths about the fascia. Before he started this journey with me, his body was big; to the untrained eye it looked great, but he was misaligned, thick, round, and in pain. It didn't take long for him to see and feel the changes once he began decompressing and strengthening the fascia. Today, he is a beautiful demonstration of a strong, aligned and healthy body.

Many people are fit but not healthy. Health and fitness require space in the tissue to receive blood and oxygen: cellular alignment. Anyone involved actively in sports will regularly be torqueing the body out of alignment in one direction. In volleyball, I was a power hitter. My practice spiking the ball with only my right arm, torqueing my body to left, allowed me to deliver an awesome blow, but, over time, twisted my body so that I experienced pain and compression and ballooning.

Balance and symmetry are the key. If every cell sits exactly where it is supposed to be, there is optimal flow. Such a body would not conventionally age. It would stay young and function with ease right up to the end. For the longest time, the scientific establishment largely ignored the fascia system. We have been taught to expect normal aging and degeneration. But it doesn't have to be this way!

Stephanie Nixon

I met Deanna and started Block Therapy over three years ago. Since then my life has genuinely changed for the amazing! Not just from having such a positive influence in my life -- she truly is one of the kindest, sweetest, and most caring (also hilarious!) people

I've met -- but from the amazing effects her system has had on my physical and mental health.

Deanna has said many times that Block Therapy is therapy, exercise and meditation all in one, and when I first heard that I really couldn't comprehend how true it was. How could one piece of wood do all that? I didn't understand that Block Therapy would be a lifestyle change and the block of wood would be just one of my tools.

I have had some pretty extreme physical and mental health issues for most, if not all, of my life. I have an auto-immune disease called Myasthenia Gravis (literally, Gravely Weak Muscles), Major Depressive Disorder, and Complex Post-Traumatic Stress Disorder. I have a few other "smaller" diagnoses, but those three are the ones that have controlled my life.

Block Therapy is the first therapy that helped me start to regain my basic muscles, after a few failed attempts with physiotherapy. I started to learn more about what my posture was doing to exacerbate the weak muscle symptoms, and cause pain elsewhere. I slowly but surely began to regain my core and stabilizing muscles. I was releasing stuck fascia and adhesions I'd developed over time as a result of horrible posture due to weak muscles.

Once I was able to support my body properly, I was shocked that I was also able to use Block Therapy as an exercise. I could do those same Block Therapy positions, but this time, by lifting or holding a leg or arm isometrically, actually **build** muscle instead of just releasing fascia. This was exciting for me, as I could go at my own pace. In the past I would try following a gym, jogging or at-home yoga routine, and would push myself too hard to keep up. I would end up having *my disease flare up, sometimes lose the ability to walk, take several days or weeks to recover, and then be back at square one, or even worse than I was to start. With Block Therapy I used the breath-as-your-guide rule and never had a flare-up of my disease.*

But the thing that surprised me most was how beneficial Block Therapy has been for my mental health. If I started to feel a panic attack coming on, I would lie in the Belly position, focus on my breathing, and the anxiety would melt away. If I was having a depressive episode and was unable to get out of bed, I would just take my Block to bed with with me. If I could accomplish one thing that day, and that was relieving some of the pain in my body with the Block, that would be enough. But more often than not I'd finish blocking in bed and that would be the baby step I needed to get out of bed and accomplish other things.

Focusing on my breath and listening to my body's pain under the Block has been key to being able to meditate for the first time in my life. My brain actually goes quiet sometimes! Still working to make it consistent, which is great, because with Block Therapy you are never truly "done". You keep finding new things to work on in order to better yourself.

I look back at myself three years ago when my days were full of pain, weakness, stress and negative self-talk. While I do still see a neurologist and psychologist and use a lot of standard medication for my auto-immune disease, Block Therapy has been the thing that tied it all together. Now I feel like a different person. I can't wait to see how far I get in the next three years!

Epilogue

A Brighter Future

Imagine a world where decompression is the health conscious focus.

People are properly aligned and able to perform physical tasks without pain. They understand how to handle stress and remove it from the body to prevent emotional and mental suffering. They have the space in mind and body to create a life filled with purpose. They are focused on the positives in work and relationship. They build community. They strive continually to improve the health of the earth and all that it houses.

Such would be a world of conscious breathers. Progress would take the form of healing and forgiveness. Everyone would be shown equal consideration, just as a conscious breather sees every cell as equal in significance. This would be a healthy world, where every decision implemented would be for the greatest good of the whole.

Fortunately, Block Therapy is on the move. The resultant ability to unlock the conscious breath and access the diaphragm to its full potential will bear gifts we can only begin to imagine. First we will decompress the fascia to shine light into old, stuck places; then we will breathe life into that space, illuminating the potentials of distant and forgotten hopes and dreams; then we will own that space, drawing our strength and determination from within. That is the fire of conscious breath. That is the driver of action.

It is my ultimate goal to share Block Therapy with all who choose to be their own health care advocates. As I said before: I knew I needed an army to get the message out. So many beautiful souls have been drawn into my life and have provided me with guidance, direction and support to continue with this mission. Everyone who has adopted and put faith in Block Therapy has enhanced my own wisdom and effectiveness.

Many look to scientific research to confirm the benefits of any new system. I look to the people who actually practise it -- who truly know. Now the benefits are undeniable, as there are thousands of practitioners, and their numbers are increasing.

If you want to be part of this community and learn more about Block Therapy from those who do it, join our private Facebook group -- Block Therapy Members -- to be part of the conversation.

Heather Mcleod Whitla

I was first introduced to Deanna Hansen's Fluid Isometrics by my Naturopath, who highly recommended her and the work that she is doing to promote health and healing. My daughter, a national Gymnast at the time, had injured her back during a practice, and she had a competition coming up that she would not be able to participate in. For at least 6 months we had been doing physiotherapy and chiropractic work with no success. I decided to take her to see Deanna, as her pain was getting worse.

After my daughter's first treatment, she walked out pain free. I was amazed; but not only that: I personally had never experienced something that overwhelmed me with such an incredible sense of "PEACE". Deanna's work on my daughter was the most beautiful "movement" I had ever seen, or felt, in my life!!

A month or so later, I contacted Deanna in hopes that she would meet with me for coffee, so that I could ask her what steps to take to have her train me in what she was doing. This seemed to me to be the missing "piece" in finding that PEACE that I had been on a lifelong quest for.

Deanna mentioned that she was in the process of closing her clinic so that she could focus on bringing Block Therapy to the world. And then she asked me the most amazing thing: would I like to help her!

I just left a marriage of 25 years and had physically succumbed to the effects of the divorce. The stress had slowly sapped my strength and will to keep going, and all of my organs had started to shut down, to the point where, had I not made it to my Naturopath, I may not have got through another day.

I was still suffering from PTSD, and struggling to stay awake long enough to get through the day, when Deanna, Block and DVD in hand, gave them to me with the instructions to "do this". This ended up being the missing link to healing my organs and broken spirit. I diligently did the entire video every day. After approximately 14 days, I started to feel an unexplainable spark of LIFE entering my body. This was the most incredible feeling, after feeling lifeless for so long. From that moment on my Block became my Magnet!! I spent every moment that I could practicing, and am alive today because of my diligence.

I am proud and honoured that Deanna Hansen has brought me on board to share my experience with the world, and to help bring Block Therapy into awareness. As one of the first two Block Therapy Instructors, I am eternally grateful for her vision of health and her trust in me.

Deanna's creation, leadership, training and devotion have provided the most inspirational "MOVEMENT" that I believe the world has ever known. I can't think of anything more incredible than this gift of LIFE!

I am so very grateful to you, Deanna, for what you have given me, and am fortunate to have this opportunity to be by your side, as *all other instructors will be, as we grow! Thank you from the bottom of my soul! We are now unveiling the "MOVEMENT" of Mind, Body, and Spirit Healing.*

About the Author

Deanna Hansen is a Certified Athletic Therapist and the founder of Fluid Isometrics and Block Therapy. She has spent over 50,000 hours working in the fascia and has seen thousands receive the transformational benefits of her system. She has a global community, along with a university program where she teaches individuals to share Block Therapy with their community.

To learn more, go to www.blocktherapy.com

Made in the USA
Monee, IL
14 March 2025